Budget Keto Kitchen

Easy recipes that are big on taste and light on the wallet

Monya Kilian Palmer

Photography by Maja Smend and Sam Folan

KYLE BOOKS

*For all my readers: I hope you can taste the love
I scatter, stir and pour into every one of my dishes.*

An Hachette UK Company
www.hachette.co.uk

First published in Great Britain in 2022 by
Kyle Books, an imprint of Octopus Publishing Group Limited
Carmelite House
50 Victoria Embankment
London EC4Y 0DZ
www.kylebooks.co.uk
www.octopusbooksusa.com

ISBN: 9781914239106

Text copyright Monya Kilian Palmer © 2022
Design and layout copyright © Octopus Publishing Group Ltd 2022
Photography copyright Maja Smend © 2022*
* except pages 23, 44–45, 49, 52, 62, 65, 66, 103, 105, 106, 112,
117, 118, 122, 127, 134–135 Sam Folan © 2022

Distributed in the US by Hachette Book Group, 1290 Avenue of the
Americas, 4th and 5th Floors, New York, NY 10104

Distributed in Canada by Canadian Manda Group, 664 Annette St.,
Toronto, Ontario, Canada M6S 2C8

Monya Kilian Palmer is hereby identified as the author of this work in
accordance with Section 77 of the Copyright, Designs and Patents Act
1988

Publisher: Joanna Copestick
Publishing Director: Judith Hannam
Editor: Tara O'Sullivan
Design: Nicky Collings
Photography: Maja Smend & Sam Folan
Food styling: Monya Kilian Palmer
Prop styling: Morag Farquhar
Production: Allison Gonsalves

A Cataloguing in Publication record for this title is available from the
British Library

Printed and bound in China

10 9 8 7 6 5 4 3 2 1

All reasonable care has been taken in the preparation of this book,
but the information it contains is not intended to take the place of
treatment by a qualified medical practitioner.

Before making any changes in your health regime, always consult
a doctor. While all the therapies detailed in this book are completely
safe if done correctly, you must seek professional advice if you are in
any doubt about any medical condition. Any application of the ideas
and information contained in this book is at the reader's sole
discretion and risk.

Contents

Introduction

Wow, here we are: book three! My loved ones are certainly not surprised, because sharing creations that are in line with a lifestyle that is so important to me is a true passion of mine, and I cannot think of a better way to do this than to inspire like-minded readers with beautiful cookbooks full of exciting, delicious recipes.

Budget Keto Kitchen is a collection of recipes inspired by a particularly vulnerable time for me. Like millions of people, the lockdowns over 2020 and 2021 were an emotionally, mentally and financially stressful period in our home. With my husband being in the entertainment industry and myself in hospitality (and both self-employed!), we were facing some challenging times. However, moving away from the ketogenic lifestyle was never even a consideration, and what resulted was probably my most enjoyable keto-related task yet: I had to get very creative, fast!

Don't get me wrong: we weren't utterly destitute and penniless, but we did have to cut down on luxuries like rib-eye steaks, wild-caught salmon, and fancy-pants almond flour. I continued to keep our meals very low in carbs, moderate in protein and high in natural fat. I ensured they were still nutrient-packed and as unprocessed as possible (processed foods are sometimes unavoidable – and there is no judgement here!).

I reached for more affordable ingredients when shopping, and often found myself raiding items forgotten at the back of the pantry. I watched my produce closely: unless it got to the point where it could grow legs and walk out the fridge on its own, I made sure it was used somehow. I dabbled in pickling and fermentation as ways to preserve fresh, half-used items (see pages 12–15), and I used leftover herbs to flavour batches of butter (pages 16–17) that I could simply melt over cooked meat or vegetables on nights I was too busy to make anything more elaborate. I also learned about shopping smart and batch-cooking.

While I am not qualified to speak about the positive psychological effect of enjoying a delicious, homemade meal at the end of a challenging day, I do know about the satisfaction a cook might feel after producing exactly that – especially on keto, where there is so much pressure to Do It Right.

I cover all the basics of living a keto lifestyle in my first two books (*Keto Kitchen* and *Lazy Keto Kitchen*), so I will not go into detail here, because I have so much more I want to share. The basics are simple: to follow a way of eating that is low in carbs and high in (natural) fat, with moderate levels of protein. Keeping those carbs consistently very low results in ketosis (the process where your body uses fat as fuel in the absence of carbohydrates). The by-products of this process are called ketones, a type of chemical produced in the liver when it breaks down fat for energy.

In this book, I wanted to show you how creative you can be with inexpensive items. If cooked and combined well, you can create a satisfying meal that everyone will simply love!

Will there be more books? You betcha! While I crack on with those, I want you to enjoy *Budget Keto Kitchen*, which has been designed to inspire you – and I hope it does just that.

– Monya

Is the Keto Lifestyle Expensive?

Great question! Before I dive in, I want to go on the record and say that sourcing grass-fed/pasture-raised, free-range, organic meat (or wild-caught, in the case of fish) will always be considered optimum. However, I would be lying if I said this was a priority of ours over the pandemic when money was a little tight. As soon as things looked up again, we did slowly return to sourcing these ingredients, as they are, ultimately, better for our overall health in the long term. I simply believe that everyone should just do the best they can within their means.

All that aside... is keto expensive? I honestly do not believe so. On a low-carb, high-fat, moderate-protein lifestyle, it is unlikely you will be eating three meals a day and snacking in between. Also, you will not be eating pricey takeaways or buying convenience foods as much. High-fat foods (especially those featuring protein) will satiate you for many hours, and you will probably start intermittent fasting without even realising it, because you are listening to your body and eating when you are hungry rather than out of habit.

A beautiful piece of cooked fatty meat will satisfy (and satiate) you for far longer than a pot of noodles will. It is also far more nutritious. Remember, too, that your blood sugar will spike after a high-carb meal, and that this will soon be followed by a crash, leaving you hungry again.

I like to think that our bodies are simply longing for something real and nutritious – and once they have it, they are satisfied. Most days of the week, my husband Mark and I only eat one meal a day (this is known as 'OMAD' in the diet-sphere). We enjoy a meal in the evenings because this is when we unwind – I find cooking very enjoyable.

Do not think of healthy food as expensive. Rather, remind yourself that unhealthy food is cheap – and no one wants to put anything 'cheap' into their bodies. It can be tricky if you are new to the keto lifestyle, but it is easier than you think – especially if you plan ahead.

Failing to Plan is Planning to Fail

One of my better qualities is that I am highly organised (although Mark may think it is more appropriate to use the word 'painfully'!). Decluttering my pantry and freezer every few months brings me so much joy. This would be the first thing I advise. Taking a quick weekly inventory of your fridge is also wise because it means you can easily plan your upcoming meals and spot any produce that needs using up.

When planning your meals and making your shopping list, take some time and look through your favourite keto recipe books, placing sticky notes on the pages that take your fancy. Review your pantry to see what dry goods you already have. Next, list the fresh items you will need. Try to choose recipes that call for the same ingredient more than once to ensure minimal wastage.

If you do not have a large freezer, take care to avoid buying more food than you need, because you will be tempted to cook it up and then, without the option of freezing it, you may unnecessarily overeat (I was guilty of this in the past!). However, if you do have freezer space, I'd suggest spending an hour or two once a week batch-cooking some handy bases, like the Beefy Mince (page 42), which can be used to make three different four-portion meals.

On that note: most meals in this book serve four, but you can easily scale up or down if needed. If you live in a smaller household, you might use your leftovers for lunch or dinner the next day. Or, of course, if you have the space, you could simply freeze your cooked portions (see page 6 for some guidance on freezing and reheating meals).

Shopping Smart

Here are my top smart shopping tips:

*

Stick to your shopping list (unless you find a particularly good bargain – see below).

*

Check the sell-by dates of meat, fish and fresh produce and choose ones that will last longer.

*

Remember that the freshest produce is not always stacked where you can see it – that's the produce they want to sell first! Reach for the back of the shelf or the rack underneath, because it will probably be marked with a later sell-by date. My *ouma* (grandmother) taught me this!

*

If you have a large freezer, check out the 'reduced to clear' shelves in your supermarket. They usually contain items whose sell-by date is that same day. Even if these items are not on your shopping list, if they suit your eating habits, grab them and pop them in your freezer, because you can still creatively use them up in the future.

This book is packed with plenty of tips and cooking techniques to help you become a confident and creative cook, so if you do go a little off-piste from your shopping list, you will still learn how to create beautiful dishes using the best asset you own: your imagination.

Special Ingredients

I have done my best to steer clear of any ingredients that may not be familiar to you. But, with keto having been around for so long, I like to think that most readers know their way around some 'special' ingredients, which can easily be sourced in health stores or online.

Arrowroot powder or ground arrowroot is found in the baking aisle. It has great thickening qualities, which makes it an essential ingredient in my Poor Man's Bourguignon (pages 107–8) and Homemade Custard (pages 128–9). It is available in little tubs, or handy 8g (¼oz) sachets (which equal 1 level tablespoon).

FREEZING, DEFROSTING & REHEATING

If you have cooked extra in order to enjoy leftovers the next day, leave the leftovers to cool a little, then cover and transfer to the fridge. Leaving it to cool a little first will prevent condensation on the lid. More importantly, it is not good practice to put anything hot inside a fridge.

If you choose to freeze cooked portions, allow the food to cool a little, then wrap up your portions (or place in suitable containers) before labelling and popping in the freezer.

The safest way to defrost items is inside the fridge overnight. With larger cuts of meat, you may need more than a day. For frozen fish or prawns, I remove them from the packaging and defrost directly on a tray lined with good-quality paper towels, because there is often an added ice-glaze that can result in your defrosted food floating in liquid.

To reheat fully defrosted meals, place them in a warm oven (120°C/100°C fan/250°F/gas mark ½) for 30–35 minutes. I find that the microwave isn't

as kind to some dishes, especially those that contain a lot of dairy: cheese or cream tends to split, and the fat runs off in different directions. While there may not be a difference in flavour, it bothers me visually.

I never freeze raw vegetables (see page 9). However, freezing a dish that includes cooked vegetables is perfectly fine.

Coconut flour is widely available online. While almond flour has always been my go-to, I have only used coconut flour in this book because it is more affordable, although in some recipes almond flour can be used instead, and I've given the quantity needed. Coconut and almond flour can't be used as direct substitutes for each other, though, and especially not in the same quantity.

Erythritol is the only natural sweetener that I use and I go for the powdered (confectioners') kind.

Ghee or lard are great stable fats to use for cooking at high temperatures in cases where regular butter is not entirely appropriate. I never use my good-quality olive oil to fry foods, and I stopped using vegetable oil years ago (I hope you have, too).

Ground (milled) chia seeds are widely available. Do not try and grind whole chia seeds yourself unless you can achieve the very fine powder the store-bought kind offers.

Inulin prebiotic powder is a store-bought soluble fibre derived from chicory root – I love it! Not only does my gut appreciate it, but it's also the only item I have found that will activate yeast in the absence of traditionally used sugar. A bag of this lasts a very long time because I never use more than a teaspoon at once. I get mine online.

Nutritional yeast flakes can be found in the same aisle as all the stocks, herbs, and spices. They boast a beautiful cheesy flavour that I need in my Nacho Beef Bowl (pages 51–3) where real cheese is not suitable.

Psyllium husk powder is an essential ingredient in all my breads and wraps: it thickens and binds a mixture like nothing else can. A bag of the powder (not husks, please) will last you a long time. Some brands of psyllium may result in a slight purple tinge in cooked goods, but this won't affect the flavour.

Nutritional Information

The nutritional breakdowns in this book were calculated using NUTRITICS® software, which is fully approved by the relevant Trading Standards organisations and is EU and FDA-compliant. I based the calculations on the trimmed weight of all the ingredients used in the recipes (apart from those shown as 'optional'). Where erythritol has been used, I have excluded its non-impact carbs.

Unless otherwise stated, I have shown the macro breakdown per serving, based on the finished dish being divided into equal-sized servings. I have stuck to moderate protein in most cases as keto suggests, but you may serve things up differently, so use the nutritional information as a guide.

Food labels differ across the world. To keep things simple, I have shown only the information that we monitor on keto: the (net) carbohydrates, proteins and fats (plus calories, for those who still count them).

Cooking Tips

I share so many great cooking tips in my first two books, so I will keep these ones short and sweet.

When I call for teaspoons or tablespoons, please get your hands on an inexpensive set of universal measuring spoons – and always level them when using dry ingredients. When a weight measurement is given, please put those spoons away – a set of kitchen scales is far more accurate.

And please don't skip salt, pepper or any freshly chopped herbs or citrus zest garnishes I call for: they are often the unsung heroes of a beautifully finished dish.

Happy cooking, everyone. You've got this!

My Keto Pantry

On this page, I've listed all the dry/pantry goods used in this book. You probably have many of them in your kitchen already. If you need to stock up, remember that a little pot of dried herbs or spices will last you a long time, so do not be disheartened if you feel a little financial pinch in your initial shop. Items like inulin powder and psyllium husk powder (two 'special' ingredients you may not be familiar with – see page 7), are also included, but only tiny amounts are used at any time, so a bag of each is well worth the small investment. Be sure to read the labels, because items like dried active yeast should be refrigerated after opening. Remember, too, that fresh basil, tomatoes, unpeeled onions, garlic and fresh ginger are best stored at room temperature, which is why I've included them here.

almond milk (unsweetened), **arrowroot powder,** Baharat spice, **baking powder,** basil (fresh), **black pepper,** brandy, capers (in brine), canned meat and fish (corned beef, salmon, tuna), caraway seeds, cardamom pods, **cayenne pepper, chilli powder,** Chinese five-spice, **cocoa powder (unsweetened), coconut flour*, coconut milk (full-fat, canned),** coconut oil (including unflavoured/odourless), coriander seeds, **curry powder,** dark chocolate (85 per cent cocoa), desiccated coconut, **dried active yeast, dried bay leaves,** dried chillies, **dried oregano,** dried sage, dry white wine, **eggs, erythritol (powdered), garlic powder,** ground allspice, **garlic,** ground (milled) chia seeds, ground cinnamon, ground coriander, ground cumin, **ground ginger,** ground nutmeg, **ground white pepper, gelatine powder, ghee,** gherkins (or cornichons), **ginger (fresh root), inulin prebiotic powder,** instant coffee, jalapeños (in brine), jarred red peppers (chargrilled), ketchup (no sugar added), liquid stevia (optional), **mayonnaise,** mustard (American-style, Dijon, wholegrain), mustard powder, mustard seeds, nutritional yeast flakes, **nuts** (flaked almonds, macadamia, mixed, pine nuts), **olive oil** (including truffle-infused), olives, **onions** (baby, regular and red), onion powder (also called onion granules), paprika, **psyllium husk powder,** ras el hanout, salt (regular, sea and flakes), **sesame oil,** sesame seeds, smoked paprika, **star anise,** sugar-free jelly powder, sugar-free syrup, **tamari, tomatoes (canned,** cherry, concentrated purée and **fresh), turmeric,** vanilla extract, **vinegar** (apple cider, balsamic, red wine, rice wine, white wine), **red wine,** Worcestershire sauce

* As you will discover, I have excluded almond flour in this book. This was because I am aware of the price difference between pricey almond 'flour' and coconut 'flour': two popular keto ingredients. I therefore worked hard to develop and perfect recipes using the latter.

My Keto Fridge

Fresh chicken, meat or fish can easily be portioned and frozen soon after purchasing. I do not advise freezing uncooked vegetables, however, because their water content will result in a soggy defrost and a bizarre, unpalatable flavour and texture. I rarely buy ready-prepped veg like courgetti or cauliflower rice: not only are they pricier than simply buying the veg and prepping it yourself, but they also have a shorter fridge-life. When it comes to frozen veg, I've never personally been a fan, because I dislike the flavour. So for me, fresh is best, and I would rather encourage you to spend a little more time (and less money) chopping, spiralising or blitzing fresh produce yourself. You will taste the difference, I promise!

asparagus, **avocado,** baby spinach, **bacon, beef** (mince, roast leftovers, steak, stewing chunks, stock), **broccoli, butter, cabbage** (red, Savoy and white), **cauliflower,** celeriac, **cheese** (Cheddar, cream, blue, feta, Gruyère, halloumi, mascarpone, mozzarella, Parmesan or Pecorino), **chicken** (drumsticks, livers, roast leftovers, stock, thighs, wings), chillies (red and green), chives, chorizo, **coriander,** courgettes, cucumber, dill, **double cream,** fennel, **fish** (any white fillets, fish pie mix, stock), ham (deli), lamb ribs, **lard,** lemon, lemongrass, lettuce/salad leaves, limes, mint, mushrooms, **parsley, pork** (belly slices, mince, roast leftovers, sausages), prawns, raspberries, red pepper, **spring onions**, soured cream, strawberries, tarragon, **thyme,** watercress, wild rocket, yellow pepper, **yogurt**

'DIRTY' KETO

There are a handful of recipes in this book where I have reached for items that are considered 'dirty' keto. This includes tasty and convenient items like chorizo, store-bought gluten-free sausages (while still very low in carbs, sausages usually contain a little added starch), tamari (a gluten-free soy sauce that many 'strict' keto followers steer clear of), no-added-sugar ketchup and sugar-free syrup.

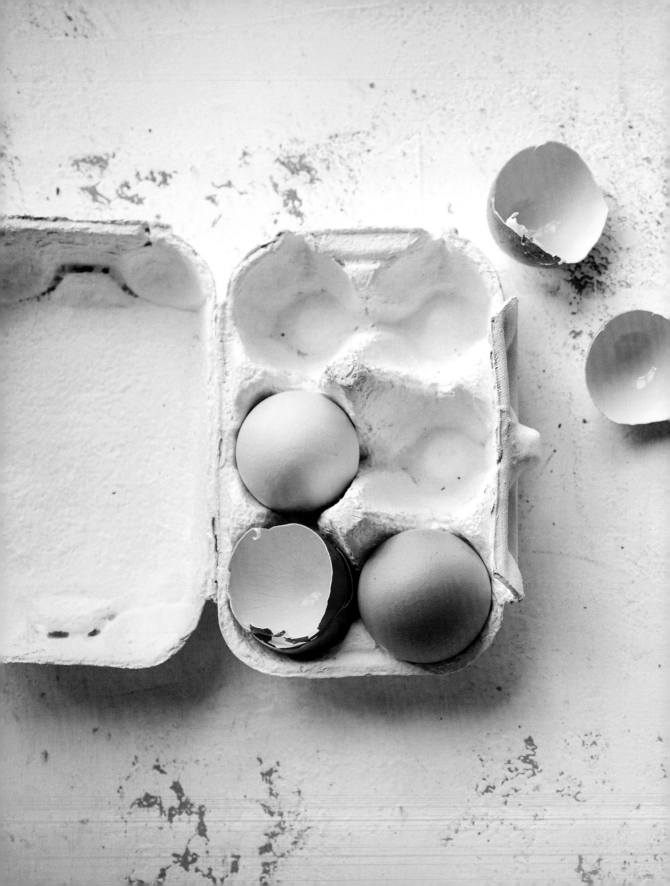

No-waste Keto

No one likes to waste fresh, unused produce, but because on keto we meticulously weigh raw ingredients, we are frequently left with half heads of cabbage or off-cuts of cauliflower and other veg. Sometimes, you might discover a lone courgette forgotten at the bottom of the fridge, or a few sad-looking half-full packets of herbs begging to be used. None of this needs to be wasted – it can still be used if you apply a little creativity.

In this chapter, I will share some easy, uncomplicated ways to use up leftover produce, from the age-old methods of pickling and fermenting, to using up wilting herbs in flavoured butters or dynamite salad dressings. I am also super excited to show you how to brown butter, which, when drizzled over vegetables or meat, can lift them to mighty levels of flavour!

We always have cauliflower kicking about in our fridge, so I'll also show you how it can be used to thicken soups, to create a versatile creamy cauliflower side, or even whipped up into a tasty paella-style dish. And let us not forget about eggs: the perfect inexpensive protein!

I've also included some fun ideas to use up leftover roast meat. Remember, if you have a large family and you don't anticipate leftovers, you could just roast two cuts (or two birds) at the same time – it will take the same amount of effort (and electricity), and means that your lazy Sunday of slow cooking could take the pressure off the first few days of the upcoming week,... and who doesn't love that convenience?

Pickles

Sharp, acidic, and often still crunchy, homemade pickles are ideal to add to salads or to serve alongside heavy, creamy dishes to cut through the richness.

Here, I've shared my Basic Pickle Mixture, along with a few different kinds of pickle to try. Have some fun and experiment: why not try pickling diced courgettes, peppers, red cabbage, baby mushrooms, or under-ripe avocados? Nothing in your fridge ever needs to go to waste.

I usually use 500ml (18fl oz) jars, but you can use larger jars if you want a bigger batch: just remember that everything should be completely submerged in the pickling liquid, and the ratio of vinegar to water should be even. Use pickling salt that contains no additives, or sea salt (which is at least non-iodised).

Basic Pickle Mixture

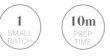

1 SMALL BATCH **10m** PREP TIME

Most vegetables will float, so fermentation weights are a useful investment to keep everything fully submerged.

120ml (4fl oz) apple cider vinegar

120ml (4fl oz) warm water (see Tip opposite)

1 teaspoon mustard seeds

1 teaspoon whole black peppercorns

2 teaspoons powdered erythritol, sifted

½ teaspoon sea salt (see above)

Combine all the ingredients in a bowl, stirring until the erythritol and salt dissolve. Set aside to cool completely before using.

Pickled Cucumber

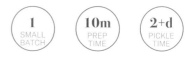

1 SMALL BATCH **10m** PREP TIME **2+d** PICKLE TIME

0.6G CARBS PER 40G (DRAINED WEIGHT)

250g (9oz) cucumber, peeled (if you prefer) and sliced

2 garlic cloves, smashed

small handful of fresh dill (or ½ teaspoon dried)

1 quantity Basic Pickle Mixture (left), cooled

Place the cucumber, garlic and dill in a clean, sterilised jar. Pour over the pickle mixture and seal. Refrigerate for at least 2 days before enjoying. These are great with my rich Nutty Cheeseburgers (page 64), or simply added to a salad for additional acidity.

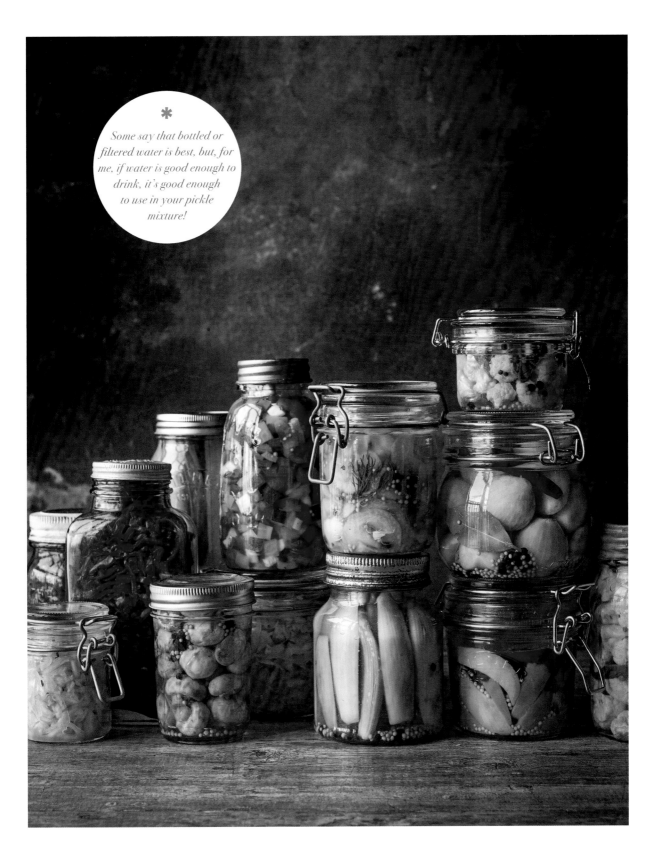

*

Some say that bottled or filtered water is best, but, for me, if water is good enough to drink, it's good enough to use in your pickle mixture!

Pickled Cauliflower

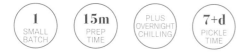

1 SMALL BATCH **15m** PREP TIME **PLUS OVERNIGHT CHILLING** **7+d** PICKLE TIME

1.2G CARBS PER 40G (DRAINED WEIGHT)

150g (5½oz) cauliflower chopped into very small florets (about 2cm/¾in)

1 quantity Basic Pickle Mixture (page 12), cooled

1 teaspoon ground turmeric

1 teaspoon toasted coriander seeds

small handful of fresh basil (leaves and stalks)

salt

Place the cauliflower in a wide-bottomed bowl and scatter generously with salt. Toss to evenly coat and leave in the fridge overnight.

The next day, rinse well in a colander under cold running water, then place in a clean, sterilised jar. Pour in the pickle mixture, along with the ground turmeric, coriander seeds and basil (fresh coriander is also lovely). Seal the jar, give it a little shake, and leave in the fridge for at least 7 days before enjoying as a quick snack. I love it in the Curried Tuna Salad (page 74) for little bursts of colourful, tasty crunch, and if you are a fan of grilled corned beef slices, this pickled cauliflower makes an excellent accompaniment.

Pickled Baby Onions

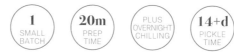

1 SMALL BATCH **20m** PREP TIME **PLUS OVERNIGHT CHILLING** **14+d** PICKLE TIME

2.8G CARBS PER 40G (DRAINED WEIGHT)

150g (5½oz) baby onions/small round shallots, peeled (see Tip on page 83 for easy peeling)

1 quantity Basic Pickle Mixture (page 12), cooled

3 dried chillies

3 dried bay leaves

salt

Place the onions in a wide-bottomed bowl and scatter generously with salt. Toss to evenly coat and leave in the fridge overnight.

The next day, rinse well in a colander under cold running water, then place in a clean, sterilised jar. Pour in the pickle mixture, along with the dried chillies and bay leaves. Seal the jar and leave in the fridge for at least 2 weeks before enjoying. These are great with cubes of strong cheese as a late-afternoon snack (Mark wanted me to add that!).

*

You could also use halved banana shallots, which are delicious when thinly sliced and tossed in a salad.

Homemade Sauerkraut

This easy fermented cabbage comes out far crunchier than the store-bought kind, and tastes deliciously fresh. I use smallish jars to ensure those half-used cabbage heads don't go to waste. The friendly bacteria that grow naturally in fermented foods are beneficial for our gut. There are just a few rules for success: clean hands, washed cabbage and sterilised jars. A non-iodised salt (sea salt) is best for fermentation, because the iodine in regular table salt inhibits the growth of the bacteria. If you are using jars with well-fitting lids, remember to open the jars for a few seconds every day to 'burp', as the gas that the bacteria produce needs to be released. *Pictured on page 13.*

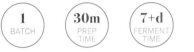

1 BATCH | 30m PREP TIME | 7+d FERMENT TIME

250g (9oz) white cabbage (trimmed weight), very thinly sliced

1 teaspoon sea salt

½ teaspoon caraway seeds

a little salted water (if needed)

Why not try this with red cabbage and a teaspoon of dried chilli flakes for a spicy red sauerkraut?

1.8G CARBS PER 40G (DRAINED WEIGHT)

Place the cabbage in a large bowl. Scatter over the salt and get stuck in with clean hands to massage the mixture, ensuring the salt is evenly distributed. Set aside for 25 minutes.

Meanwhile, toast the caraway seeds in a small non-stick pan over a medium–high heat for about 30 seconds until fragrant. Remove from the heat and add to the bowl of cabbage, mixing well to combine.

Pack the cabbage mixture down into a sterilised 500ml (18fl oz) jar, ensuring it is pushed down and compacted. You will notice some excess moisture leaching from the cabbage in the bowl. Do not discard this – in fact, you want this liquid to cover the compacted cabbage. If your cabbage doesn't produce enough liquid, add a dash of salted water to the jar. Cut a small circle of baking paper and place it on top of the cabbage, then top this with a fermentation weight. Press down to ensure all the cabbage is submerged. Close the lid, and leave in a cool, dark place for around 7 days, checking in on it once a day (see above). You will notice some foam and froth; this is a good sign.

After 7 days, it should smell deliciously sour and will be ready to eat. The jar can then be transferred to the fridge, where your sauerkraut should last a long time (although I dip in every time I walk past the fridge, so I can't say it lasts very long in our house!).

Compound Butters

Making a delicious, flavoured butter is a great way to use up leftover herbs or even pantry spices. I use the Curry Butter in Mum's Curry & Rice (page 46) and the Caramelised Sweet Onion Butter in my Mini Pork Sliders (page 67). The other ideas can be used however you like to bring a little flavour and interest to your meals: simply melt them over grilled meats, fish or even vegetables. You could even tuck a slice or two under the skin of chicken thighs before cooking. I also like to melt some slices into cooked cauliflower rice.

You will notice I refer to using softened butter: this is simply butter that has been left at room temperature for several hours, making it easier to combine with your chosen mixtures.

The carbs indicated are based on one sliced disc, assuming each log is sliced into 6 even slices.

GARLIC & PARSLEY BUTTER

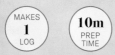

MAKES **1** LOG

10m PREP TIME

0.5G CARBS PER 15G SLICE

75g (2¾oz) unsalted butter, softened

2 garlic cloves, crushed with a garlic press

generous handful of fresh flat-leaf parsley leaves, finely chopped (approx. 5g/¹⁄₈oz)

generous pinch of salt flakes

Combine the ingredients in a bowl until well mixed together, then tip out on to a square of clingfilm. Use the clingfilm to help you shape and roll the butter mixture into a fat log, approximately 3.5cm (1¼in) in diameter and 9cm (3½in) long. Twist the ends of the clingfilm and transfer to the fridge (or freezer) until needed (it will keep for up to 1 week in the fridge). Remove from the fridge 10–20 minutes before slicing and using.

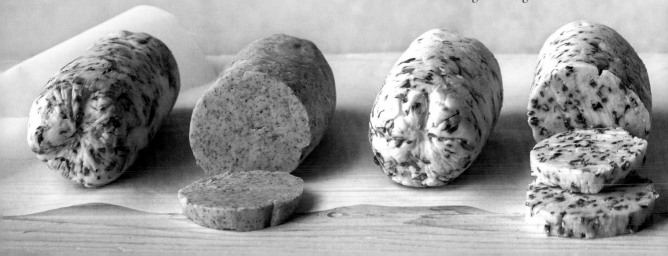

'BÉARNAISE' BUTTER

 MAKES **1** LOG   **10m** PREP TIME

<0.5G CARBS PER 15G SLICE

75g (2¾oz) unsalted butter, softened

1 teaspoon white wine vinegar

generous handful of fresh tarragon leaves, finely chopped (approx. 5g/¹/₈oz)

generous pinch of salt flakes

Follow the same method as for the Garlic & Parsley Butter.

CURRY BUTTER

MAKES **1** LOG   **5m** PREP TIME

<0.5G CARBS PER 13G SLICE

75g (2¾oz) unsalted butter, softened

1½ teaspoons curry powder

generous pinch of salt flakes

Follow the same method as for the Garlic & Parsley Butter.

CARAMELISED SWEET ONION BUTTER

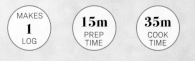 MAKES **1** LOG   **15m** PREP TIME   **35m** COOK TIME

1.1G CARBS PER 15G SLICE

75g (2¾oz) unsalted butter, softened

½ onion, finely chopped

1 tablespoon white wine vinegar

generous pinch of salt flakes

Melt 2 teaspoons of the softened butter in a very small, non-stick pan over a low heat. Add the onion and cook for 25 minutes until completely softened. Add the vinegar and continue to cook for 5 minutes, or until the onion starts to darken and caramelise and there is no moisture in the pan.

Set aside to cool a little before combining with the remaining butter using the same method as in the previous recipes.

LEMON & THYME BUTTER

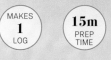 MAKES **1** LOG   **15m** PREP TIME

0.5G CARBS PER 13G SLICE

75g (2¾oz) unsalted butter, softened

finely grated zest of 1 lemon

generous handful of fresh thyme, leaves picked and finely chopped (approx. 5g/¹/₈oz)

generous pinch of salt flakes

Follow the same method as for the Garlic & Parsley Butter.

*

Have some fun: play around with smoked paprika or turmeric, or why not try grated Parmesan with plenty of snipped chives?

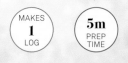

Browned Butter

(Your New Best Friend)

MAKES **200g**

15m COOK TIME

2+h SETTING TIME

250g (9oz) unsalted butter

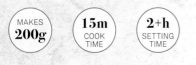

FOR GARLIC-INFUSED BROWNED BUTTER

Add 7–8 smashed garlic cloves to the pan with the butter and follow the same method as for regular browned butter. There may be more bubbles present due to the moisture in the garlic, so the butter may take longer to brown. Discard the garlic along with the milk solids when you strain.

Let's take butter up a notch! The French call this *beurre noisette*, and it is not only heavenly (with a deeply rich, nutty flavour and an aroma not unlike caramel), but it is also dead easy to make. It can be used to cook eggs, or you can add it to your baking or melt it over cooked meat and vegetables. And yet more good news: since the straining process essentially removes the milk solids, browned butter is even lower in carbs than regular butter). If you love it (and I know you will), this will become your new favourite go-to!

PER 20G SERVING:

CALORIES 176 | CARBS 0G | FAT 20G | PROTEIN 0G

Melt the butter in a large saucepan over a medium heat. Once completely melted, increase the heat to high and keep an eye on the pan. You will see the butter soon starts foaming, then bubbling. Keep stirring with a small silicone spatula, and you will notice a delicious caramel aroma as the milk solids sink and start browning. The butter itself will become dark golden.

Strain the melted butter into a bowl through a sieve lined with a double layer of food-grade muslin or cheesecloth. Discard the cloth and all the browned milk solids, then pour the strained butter into a suitably-sized tray or wide-bottomed bowl (I recommend you line it with a sheet of baking paper for easier removal). Allow to cool a little, then transfer to the fridge for several hours to set.

Once set, slice the butter into handy little blocks of approximately 20g (¾oz) pieces, which you can grab with ease when cooking. These blocks can be kept in the fridge, or wrapped up and frozen.

Lift Your Greens Game!

CABBAGE & SPINACH IN BROWNED BUTTER

SERVES 4 AS A SIDE DISH AT 2.8G CARBS PER SERVING

Melt 60g (2¼oz) Browned Butter or Garlic-infused Browned Butter in a large non-stick pan over a medium heat. Add 200g (7oz) thinly sliced cabbage and fry for 10–12 minutes until softened. Add 200g (7oz) baby spinach leaves and cook until the spinach wilts. Stir in 50g (1¾oz) soured cream and warm through, seasoning generously with salt and pepper.

VEG 'RICE' MEDLEY IN BROWNED BUTTER

SERVES 4 AS A SIDE DISH AT 3.2G CARBS PER SERVING

Blitz 160g (5¾oz) each of cauliflower, broccoli and courgettes in a food processor. Melt 60g (2¼oz) Browned Butter or Garlic-infused Browned Butter in a large non-stick pan over a medium heat and fry the veg for 14–15 minutes until softened, stirring regularly. Season with salt and pepper.

CELERIAC IN GARLIC-INFUSED BROWNED BUTTER

SERVES 4 AS A SIDE DISH AT 2.9G CARBS PER SERVING

Bring a large pan of salted water to the boil and cook 500g (1lb 2oz) peeled celeriac (diced into 1cm/½in pieces) for about 10 minutes until tender. Drain well in a colander and allow to steam off completely on a large tray lined with paper towels. Melt 40g (1½oz) Garlic-infused Browned Butter in a large non-stick pan or wok over a medium heat and add the celeriac. Fry until the pieces are browned on the outside and tender on the inside (this can take 18–20 minutes). Season with salt and pepper.

Brown-buttered Halloumi Fingers

Everyone loves halloumi 'fries' (and many pubs now offer them, which is great for those living low carb!). However, I wanted to try using the luxurious flavour of my Browned Butter (page 18) to cook batons of this delicious squeaky cheese. These are so yummy simply dipped in a little no-added-sugar ketchup. This serves 4 people as a side dish or a little appetiser, but they're also great in the salad below.

CALORIES 408 | CARBS 0.9G | FAT 35G | PROTEIN 22G

4 SERVINGS | **5m** PREP TIME | **5m** COOK TIME

40g (1½oz) Browned Butter (page 18)

400g (14oz) full-fat halloumi cheese, drained and sliced

salt flakes (optional)

*

Steer clear of reduced-fat halloumi if possible: I find it crumbles more.

You may need to cook these in batches. Melt the browned butter in a large non-stick pan or wok over a medium–high heat and gently fry the halloumi slices until golden on all sides. Transfer to a plate lined with paper towels to drain. Season with salt flakes only if needed (halloumi tends to be quite salty already).

Avocado & Halloumi Salad

This beautiful salad is really all about easy, clever seasoning: good-quality olive oil, zesty lemon and lovely, fresh ingredients. I've topped it with the Brown-buttered Halloumi Fingers (above), making it a surprisingly filling meal, especially in the summer months.

CALORIES 609 | CARBS 5.6G | FAT 53G | PROTEIN 24G

4 SERVINGS | **20m** PREP TIME | **5m** COOK TIME

2 large avocados, cut into chunks

1 red pepper, finely diced

½ red onion, very thinly sliced

generous squeeze of fresh lemon juice

160g (5¾oz) cherry tomatoes, halved

2 tablespoons olive oil

70g (2½ oz) baby spinach leaves

1 quantity Brown-buttered Halloumi Fingers (see above)

salt and freshly ground black pepper

Place the avocado, red pepper and red onion in a bowl. Squeeze over the lemon juice (catch the pips!) and toss to combine. Season with black pepper, then cover and set aside in the fridge until needed.

In a separate bowl, combine the cherry tomatoes and olive oil, seasoning with salt flakes. Cover and set aside at room temperature until needed.

When ready to serve, simply combine all the elements and serve over the baby spinach. Top with the fried halloumi fingers.

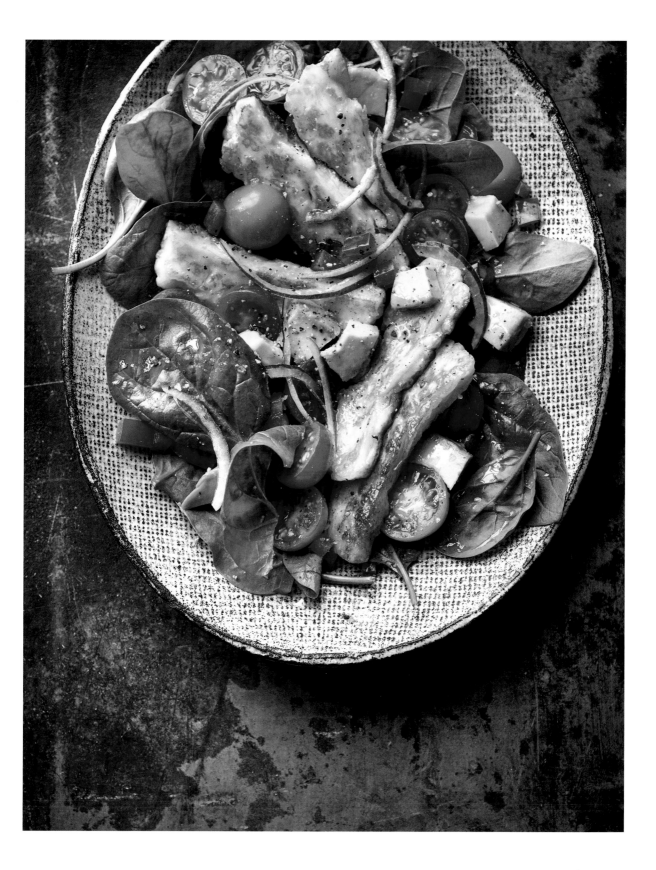

Crustless Quiche Lorraine

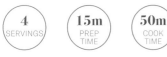

4 SERVINGS

15m PREP TIME

50m COOK TIME

Celebrating eggs! This easy, decadent crustless quiche features smoked bacon lardons in a lightly cheese-flavoured savoury set 'custard'. It can be sliced into 8 if you prefer, but the carbs are so low that one quiche is suitable for 4 people to share. If you enjoy it with a lovely acidic salad on the side, you will have a fantastically rich and satisfying meal. *Pictured here with Mushroom & Cheese Soufflé Omelette (see page 24) and Cheese & Herb Omelette (see page 25).*

CALORIES 558 | CARBS 3.5G | FAT 52G | PROTEIN 20G

1 teaspoon unsalted butter

200g (7oz) smoked bacon lardons

3 large eggs

180ml (6fl oz) double cream

75g (2¾oz) soured cream

75g (2¾oz) full-fat cream cheese

60g (2¼oz) full-fat mature Cheddar cheese, finely grated

ground white pepper

small handful of fresh chives, snipped, to garnish (optional)

✳

Eggs are notorious for sticking to even the best-quality non-stick tins. I use the back of a teaspoon to nudge the sides of the tin, making it easy for the whole quiche to be lifted out and sliced.

Preheat the oven to 200°C/180°C fan/400°F/gas mark 6 and grease an 18cm (7in) loose-bottomed tart tin. Line the base (and a little way up the sides) with baking paper, then place the tin on a baking tray. (Letting the baking paper come up the sides just a little helps avoid the mixture leaking out the bottom, which can often happen with loose-bottomed tart tins.)

Melt the butter in a non-stick pan or wok over a medium heat and cook the bacon lardons for 8-10 minutes until they release all their moisture and are safely cooked through. Do not allow them to crisp for this recipe. Remove and set aside to cool a little.

In a mixing bowl, whisk together the eggs, double cream, soured cream and cream cheese until the mixture is smooth with no lumps. Add the Cheddar and the slightly cooled bacon bits. Season with a generous pinch of ground white pepper and mix well to combine. Pour into the prepared tin.

Keep the tin on the baking tray and bake for 25 minutes (rotating the tray halfway through to ensure even baking), then turn the oven off. Leave the oven door slightly open and leave the quiche in there for another 15 minutes to gently finish cooking through in the residual heat.

Once done, remove the quiche from the oven and leave on a cooling rack to cool a little. Scatter over snipped chives before slicing and serving (see Tip) if you want to be a little fancy. This quiche is packed with enormous, rich flavours, but Mark loves it with a dash of hot sauce!

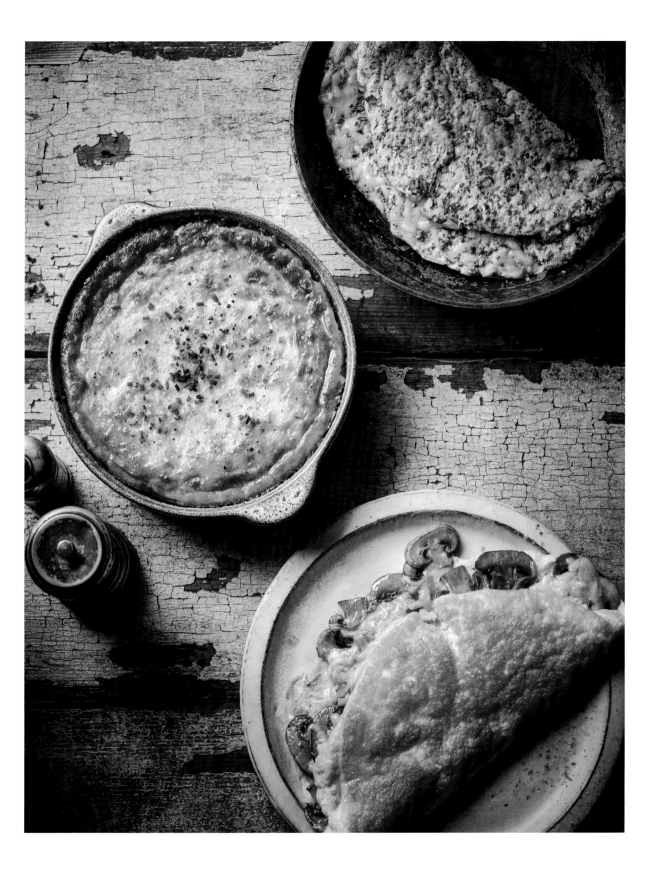

Mushroom & Cheese Soufflé Omelette

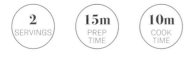

2 SERVINGS

15m PREP TIME

10m COOK TIME

2 tablespoons unsalted butter

150g (5½oz) mushrooms, sliced

3 large eggs, separated

60g (2¼oz) full-fat mature Cheddar cheese, grated

salt and freshly ground black pepper

✳

An excellent-quality pan free of rust and scratches will ensure the eggs don't stick or burn.

For this soufflé omelette, I have used caramelised mushrooms, but any leftover cooked vegetables will work a treat. Consider finely chopping leftover peppers and onions and cooking them up for a lovely veggie-packed meal. This recipe will make one large omelette, and the macros are shown per half omelette, as it is great shared between two people with a lovely fresh salad on the side. Double up the ingredients and repeat the method to make a second omelette if you want to serve four. *Pictured on page 23.*

PER ½ OMELETTE

CALORIES 356 | CARBS 3.4G | FAT 30G | PROTEIN 20G

Melt 1 tablespoon of the butter in a large non-stick pan or wok over a medium–high heat. Add the mushrooms and fry for 4–5 minutes or until they release all their moisture and start to caramelise. Remove and set aside on a plate lined with paper towels. Season with salt.

Place the egg yolks in a medium bowl and season with salt and pepper. Lightly whisk to break them up. Place the egg whites in a second, larger bowl, and use a hand mixer to whip them to stiff peaks. Add the yolks to the bowl of whites and gently fold in, retaining as much air as possible.

Wipe clean the pan you used for the mushrooms and melt the remaining 1 tablespoon butter over a medium heat. Pour in the fluffy egg mixture, smoothing the top gently with a silicone spatula. Cover with a lid or some foil and leave to cook for 1 minute, then slide your spatula around the edges to loosen any parts that may be sticking. Scatter the cooked mushrooms over half of the omelette and top with grated cheese. Cover once more and leave for another minute.

Slide a large spatula underneath the omelette and fold the omelette in half. Cover and leave for another minute before serving, although you may be able to judge by sight if your eggs are cooked through, in which case serve immediately.

Cheese & Herb Omelette

This omelette doesn't require any fancy fillings, because the predominant flavour comes from a selection of mixed herbs. Use whichever soft herbs you have on hand (see Tip), but I think coriander, parsley and chives work beautifully here. You may be able to smash through one omelette by yourself, but I like to split one between two people because it is so rich thanks to the cheese! Double up the ingredients and repeat the method to make a second omelette if you want to serve four. *Pictured on page 23.*

2 SERVINGS | **15m** PREP TIME | **10m** COOK TIME

3 large eggs

½ teaspoon garlic powder

very generous handful of fresh coriander leaves, finely chopped

very generous handful of fresh flat-leaf parsley leaves, finely chopped

very generous handful of fresh chives, finely snipped

1 tablespoon unsalted butter

50g (1¾oz) mozzarella, grated

20g (¾oz) Parmesan or Pecorino cheese, finely grated

salt and freshly ground black pepper

PER ½ OMELETTE

CALORIES 289 | CARBS 2.4G | FAT 22G | PROTEIN 20G

In a medium bowl, whisk together the eggs, garlic powder and all the herbs. Season with salt and pepper.

Melt the butter in a large, good-quality non-stick pan (see Tip opposite) over a medium heat. Pour in the egg mixture and cover with a lid or some foil. Leave to cook for 1 minute, then slide a silicone spatula around the edges to loosen parts that may stick.

Scatter the mozzarella and Parmesan over one half of the omelette, then slide a large spatula underneath the omelette and fold it in half. Cover and leave for another 45 seconds–1 minute before serving, although you may be able to judge by sight if your eggs are cooked through, in which case serve immediately.

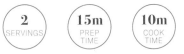

Soft herbs are exactly that: their leaves are soft and their flavour is milder than herbs with woodier stalks like rosemary, thyme, sage and bay.

Cauliflower Cheese Soup

with Loads of Bacon (obvs)

This simple, tasty soup is made using cauliflower, stock, Cheddar and plenty of smoked bacon. It is simple, hearty and surprisingly filling. It's also low enough in carbs to enjoy with your favourite buttered keto rolls, like those on page 71 or page 108. *Pictured here with Hearty Fish Chowder (see page 28).*

4 SERVINGS | **10m** PREP TIME | **25m** COOK TIME

CALORIES 577 | CARBS 4.7G | FAT 50G | PROTEIN 27G

1 tablespoon unsalted butter

200g (7oz) smoked streaky bacon, finely chopped (see Tip)

1 litre (1¾ pints) chicken stock

500g (1lb 2oz) cauliflower, chopped into small, even-sized pieces

pinch of grated nutmeg

160g (5¾oz) full-fat mature Cheddar cheese, grated

150ml (5fl oz/¼ pint) double cream

salt, ground white pepper and freshly ground black pepper

generous handful of fresh flat-leaf parsley, finely chopped, to garnish

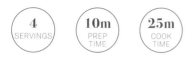

Putting the bacon in the freezer for 30 minutes before chopping will make it much easier to cut into smaller pieces. Alternatively, you can use smoked bacon lardons.

Melt the butter in a large non-stick frying pan over a medium–high heat. Add the bacon pieces and fry for 8–10 minutes until golden and crispy. Use a slotted spoon to remove the bacon pieces from the pan and set them aside on a plate to keep warm. Do not discard the rendered fat left in the pan.

In a large saucepan, bring the chicken stock to the boil and add the cauliflower. Cover with a lid and simmer over a medium heat for 15–18 minutes until the cauliflower completely softens. Pierce a floret with a fork – it should immediately slide off. Pour in the rendered fat from the bacon pan, then add the nutmeg. Use a hand blender, right there in the pan, to blitz everything to a smooth consistency, ensuring the bacon fat emulsifies into the warm mixture. If it feels far too thick, add a dash of water. If you feel it's too thin, leave on the heat a little longer to reduce further.

Once you are happy with the soup's consistency, stir in most of the grated cheese, along with most of the bacon pieces and the double cream, keeping the pan over a low heat so everything can warm through. Season with a little salt and white pepper (but remember the smoked bacon will add plenty of saltiness).

Divide the soup between 4 bowls and scatter over the remaining grated cheese and bacon. Finish with a scattering of chopped parsley, then season with salt flakes and freshly ground black pepper (if needed) before serving.

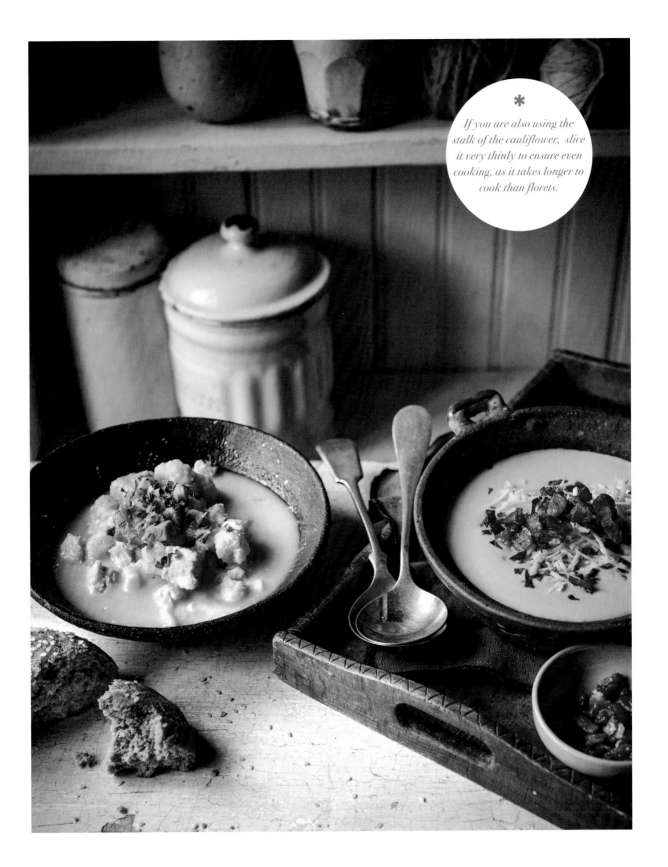

*

If you are also using the stalk of the cauliflower, slice it very thinly to ensure even cooking, as it takes longer to cook than florets.

Hearty Fish Chowder

There are several stages to this recipe, but I have my reasons! The flavours are so dreamy and comforting. I like to blitz half the cooked cauliflower to add some 'body' to the soup, then use the remaining cauliflower to add the chunky texture. I use a convenient 'fish pie mix' here (available in most UK supermarkets), but if you cannot find it, use equal amounts of skinned smoked haddock, salmon, and white fish, all cut into small pieces for even cooking. Remember: when buying any store-bought stock, take some time to check the labels, because many contain sugar and added starch. *Pictured on page 27.*

4 SERVINGS | **20m** PREP TIME | **40m** COOK TIME

CALORIES 489 | CARBS 8.1G | FAT 32G | PROTEIN 40G

1 litre (1¾ pints) fish stock

200ml (7fl oz) water

500g (1lb 2oz) cauliflower, chopped into small, even-sized pieces

1 dried bay leaf

200g (7oz) smoked bacon lardons

2 tablespoons unsalted butter

1 onion, finely diced

2 garlic cloves, finely diced

60ml (4 tablespoons) dry white wine

450g (1lb) fish pie mix

pinch of ground nutmeg

3 tablespoons double cream

salt and ground white pepper

To finish

finely grated zest of 1 lemon

small handful of fresh flat-leaf parsley leaves, finely chopped

✳

Remember, the bacon is salty, so season with salt only if you feel it is needed.

In a large saucepan with a well-fitting lid, combine the fish stock and water and bring to the boil. Add the cauliflower and bay leaf, then cover and leave to simmer over a medium–high heat for 18–20 minutes until the cauliflower is tender. Remove the pan from the heat and use a slotted spoon to remove half of the cooked cauliflower florets, setting them aside in a bowl for now. Remove and discard the bay leaf, then set this pan and its contents aside.

Meanwhile, place a large non-stick frying pan or wok over a medium heat. Add the bacon lardons and fry for 8–9 minutes until cooked through and almost crispy. Remove with a slotted spoon and set aside on a plate. Reduce the heat to low, then melt the butter in the same pan. Add the onion and garlic and cook for 8–10 minutes until completely softened. Increase the heat to high and add the white wine; this will deglaze the pan. Once all the wine has evaporated, scrape the cooked onion and garlic into the soup mixture in the other pan.

Use a hand blender, right there in the pan, to blitz the mixture until smooth. Place the pan over a medium heat and bring to a light simmer. Add the fish pie mix, along with a pinch of ground nutmeg, and leave to cook for 12–13 minutes to allow the fish to sufficiently cook through, stirring occasionally. Return the reserved cooked cauliflower to the pan, along with half the reserved cooked bacon. Add the cream and warm the chowder through. Taste and adjust the seasoning with ground white pepper (see Tip).

To serve, divide between 4 warm bowls and scatter over the remaining bacon bits, along with the lemon zest and chopped parsley.

Creamy Cauliflower Rice

Like many of you, I have made cauliflower rice, cauliflower mash and cauliflower couscous – and I love them all! Here, I wanted to play around with the flavour of the mash, but still retain a little texture – and I think this version is now my favourite! I had no idea what to title it, but 'creamy cauliflower rice' seemed to be the most accurate. Enjoy it as a base for any saucy dish – and get creative folding through different herbs and spices, or one of my flavoured butters (pages 16–17) to complement and enhance the flavour of the meal you are serving it with. *Pictured on page 85.*

4 SERVINGS | **15m** PREP TIME | **10m** COOK TIME

CALORIES 370 | CARBS 5.4G | FAT 36G | PROTEIN 6G

500g (1lb 2oz) cauliflower florets, chopped into small, even-sized pieces

40g (1½oz) unsalted butter

70g (2½oz) full-fat cream cheese

180ml (6fl oz) double cream

herbs or spices of your choice, or 2–3 slices of your chosen Compound Butter from pages 16–17 (optional)

salt and ground white pepper

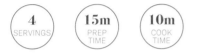

Like any recipe, the size of the pan you use will affect cooking times on the hob, as will increasing or decreasing ingredient amounts.

Blitz the cauliflower in a mini food processor or food chopper until it resembles coarse breadcrumbs. You may need to do this in batches if your food processor is as small as mine.

Melt the butter in a large non-stick pan or wok over a medium heat and add the cauliflower 'rice'. Cook for 5–6 minutes, stirring regularly, until it starts to soften (see Tip). (If you decide to enhance your mixture with a ground spice, add it now to allow the spice to cook out.)

Add the cream cheese and cream, stirring well to combine. Reduce the heat to low and continue to stir for 4–5 minutes until you are left with a thick, creamy mixture. Season generously with salt and ground white pepper.

Before serving, stir through any herbs or flavoured butter you have chosen.

Monnie's 'Paella'

I just love this 'paella', where I literally throw in everything I can find! There are two tips I would like to share here: one is to use a cartouche (a handy technique if you only want to partially allow evaporation while simmering a mixture), and the second is to slice your prawns in half lengthways. I once saw this done in a salad I'd ordered in a restaurant. I assumed they were trying to give patrons the impression that they were getting more prawns than there actually were. At the time, I thought, 'What a cheek!'. However, now I think it's pure genius!

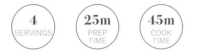

4 SERVINGS | **25m** PREP TIME | **45m** COOK TIME

CALORIES 390 | CARBS 7.4G | FAT 23G | PROTEIN 36G

2 tablespoons lard or ghee

340g (11¾oz) skinless, deboned chicken breasts (or thighs), chopped into bite-sized pieces

120g (4¼oz) uncooked, shelled prawns, halved lengthways

2 tablespoons unsalted butter

500g (1lb 2oz) cauliflower florets, blitzed into 'rice' (see page 29 for instructions)

2 garlic cloves, finely chopped

2 teaspoons smoked paprika

½ teaspoon ground turmeric

85g (3oz) chorizo, chopped into small pieces

300ml (10fl oz) chicken stock

2 tomatoes, chopped

finely grated zest and juice of 1 lemon

handful of fresh flat-leaf parsley leaves, finely chopped

salt and freshly ground black pepper

Melt 1½ tablespoons of your chosen fat in a large non-stick pan or wok over a high heat. Add the chicken pieces and fry for 3–4 minutes or until caramelised on the outside. Remove with a slotted spoon or tongs and set aside in a bowl. This is best done in a couple of batches to avoid overcrowding your pan. An overcrowded pan may prevent caramelisation. Don't worry about whether they're completely cooked through; they will simmer further later.

Add the remaining ½ tablespoon of fat to the pan and add the prawns, frying for less than a minute, or just until they turn pink. You will notice they curl up because of how we sliced them – which looks super cute! Remove from the pan and set aside in a separate bowl.

At this stage, I like to switch to using butter! Reduce the heat to medium and add the butter to the same pan you used for the chicken and prawns. Add the cauliflower 'rice', garlic, paprika and turmeric, and mix well to evenly coat the cauliflower. Cook for 4–5 minutes, stirring continuously.

Now add the chorizo and chicken stock to the pan. Cover with a cartouche (a circular piece of baking paper cut to the same diameter as your pan and placed directly on the mixture). Leave to simmer for 10 minutes, then discard the cartouche. Return the chicken pieces (including any resting juices) to the pan, along with the tomatoes. Simmer, uncovered, for 5 minutes more, adding the prawns at the last minute to gently reheat them without overcooking. Taste and adjust the seasoning with salt and pepper as needed.

Just before serving, stir in the lemon zest and juice (catch the pips!) and scatter over the parsley.

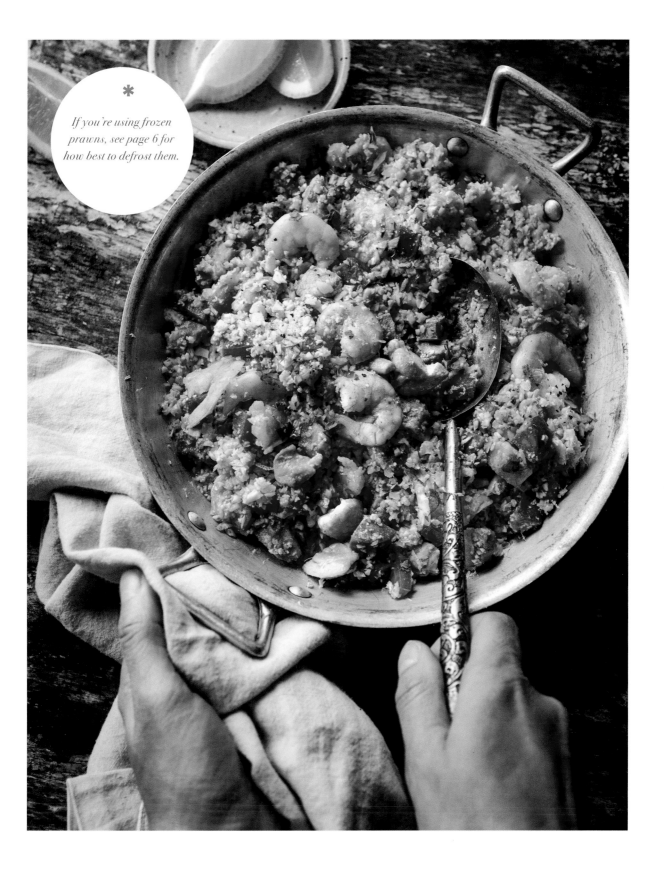

*

If you're using frozen prawns, see page 6 for how best to defrost them.

Parmesan, Rocket & Asparagus Salad

Here is a fresh idea for Mondays or Tuesdays when you need to use up slices of Sunday's roast beef. You will see I call for Parmesan cheese, but Pecorino can also be used. Just so you know, I went to a cheese seminar several years ago and learned that Parmesan (if wrapped well), gets even better in flavour the longer it is kept in the fridge: this is a win-win for Parmesan-lovers! Please note that the times indicated here exclude the actual roasting of the beef. *Pictured on page 35.*

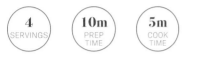

4 SERVINGS | **10m** PREP TIME | **5m** COOK TIME

CALORIES 365 | CARBS 1G | FAT 26G | PROTEIN 31G

180g (6½oz) asparagus, trimmed and sliced (trimmed weight)

60g (2¼oz) wild rocket

4 tablespoons olive oil

320g (11¼oz) leftover roast beef, thinly sliced

40g (1½oz) Parmesan or Pecorino cheese, shaved

freshly squeezed lemon juice (optional)

salt and freshly ground black pepper

Bring a small saucepan of salted water to the boil and add the asparagus, cooking for no longer than 2–3 minutes (depending on how thick they are). Drain, then plunge into a bowl of iced water. Once cooled, drain well and set aside.

Place the rocket in a bowl and drizzle over half the olive oil. Season with a little salt and toss lightly to evenly coat. Serve with the beef pieces and asparagus, then top with the shavings of cheese. Drizzle over the remaining olive oil and finish with a generous crack of black pepper. You may enjoy a little acidity with this salad, in which case you can squeeze over a little lemon juice.

OTHER IDEAS FOR USING UP LEFTOVER ROAST BEEF

Generously spread a full batch of Ranch Dressing Dip (page 89) over 4 Soft Tortilla Wraps (page 72). Divide 300g (10½oz) leftover roast beef slices, 200g (7oz) thinly sliced tomatoes, and 30g (1oz) wild rocket between each one before wrapping up!

MAKES 4 WRAPS AT 8.2G CARBS PER WRAP

Fry 2 tablespoons store-bought red curry paste in a large non-stick frying pan. Add 400g (14oz) can full-fat coconut milk and cook until the mixture thickens and reduces by more than half. Add 350g (12oz) leftover roast beef (chopped or sliced) and warm through before serving over a base like cooked courgetti. Scatter over some chopped coriander.

MAKES 4 SERVINGS AT 5.3G CARBS PER SERVING (EXCLUDING COURGETTI)

For a tasty stir-fry, finely chop 2 garlic cloves, 10g (¼oz) fresh ginger, 1 red chilli and fry with 300g (10½oz) sliced mushrooms in 1 tablespoon coconut oil. Once softened, add 350g (12oz) cooked beef slices and warm through. Finish with 1 tablespoon tamari, a squeeze of lime and a scattering of fresh coriander. Delicious over cooked cauliflower rice.

MAKES 4 SERVINGS AT 3G CARBS PER SERVING (EXCLUDING CAULI RICE)

Pulled Pork Burgers

This recipe uses leftover pork shoulder (or leg), which can easily be pulled into smaller shreds while warm. Please note that the times indicated exclude the cooking of the pork or the making of the burger buns. However, the macros do include the Whole Lot. *Pictured on page 34.*

4 SERVINGS

20m PREP TIME

1+h PICKLE TIME

5m COOK TIME

CALORIES 487 | CARBS 8.9G | FAT 34G | PROTEIN 36G

120g (4¼oz) no-added-sugar ketchup

1½ tablespoons Worcestershire sauce

½ tablespoon smoked paprika

¾ teaspoon powdered erythritol, sifted

½ teaspoon mustard powder

½ teaspoon garlic powder

½ teaspoon ground ginger

300g (10½oz) cooked roast pork leftovers, pulled (see Tip)

salt and freshly ground black pepper

For the pickled cabbage

120g (4¼oz) red cabbage, thinly sliced

90ml (6 tablespoons) red wine vinegar

60g (2¼oz) soured cream

To finish

generous handful of wild rocket

1 teaspoon olive oil

4 Burger Buns (page 71)

✳

To 'pull' cooked pork, use 2 forks on warm meat to shred into very thin strands. Follow the direction of the meat's grain (how the muscle fibres are aligned).

Start with the pickled cabbage. Simply combine the shredded cabbage with the red wine vinegar in a bowl and set aside in the fridge. Give it a stir every now and then to ensure even pickling. I like to leave mine for at least an hour, but the longer, the better, so you could make this the day before if you have the time.

To make the pork mixture, combine the ketchup, Worcestershire sauce, smoked paprika, erythritol, mustard powder, garlic powder and ground ginger in a bowl. Season with salt and pepper. Place the mixture in a large non-stick frying pan or wok and bring to a light simmer over a medium heat. Reduce the heat to low and tip in the shredded pork. Leave to warm through for 1–2 minutes until you are ready to assemble your burgers.

To finish, lightly dress the rocket leaves with olive oil and season with salt. Drain the cabbage (discarding the vinegar) and stir through the soured cream. Divide the rocket between the bun halves and pile on the warm pulled pork mixture, followed by the hot-pink cabbage. Finish with the bun top – lush!

OTHER IDEAS FOR USING UP LEFTOVER ROAST PORK

Combine pulled pork with some mayonnaise and a little wholegrain mustard for a delicious filling for the Mini Bread Rolls on page 108 or the Soft Tortilla Wraps on page 72!

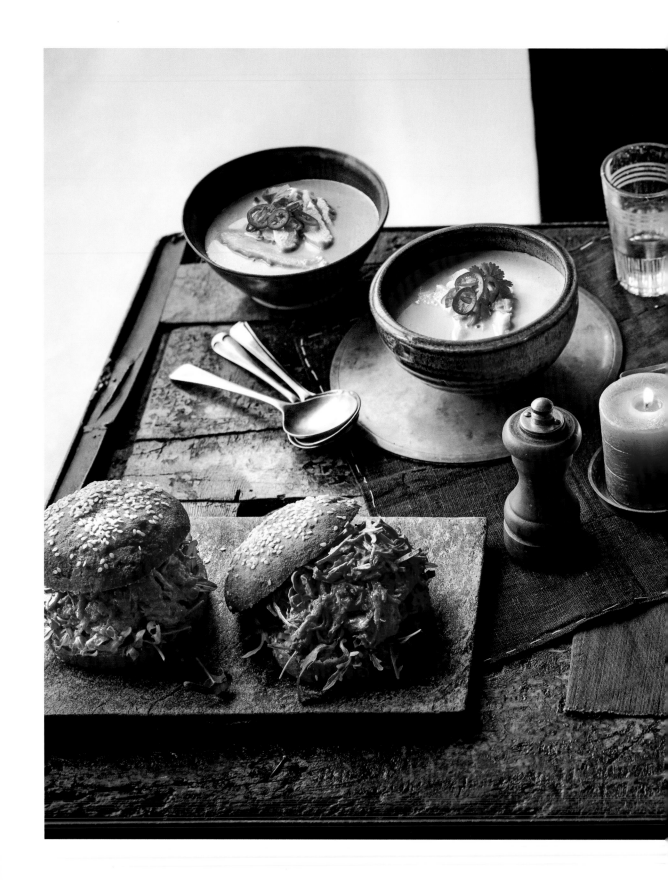

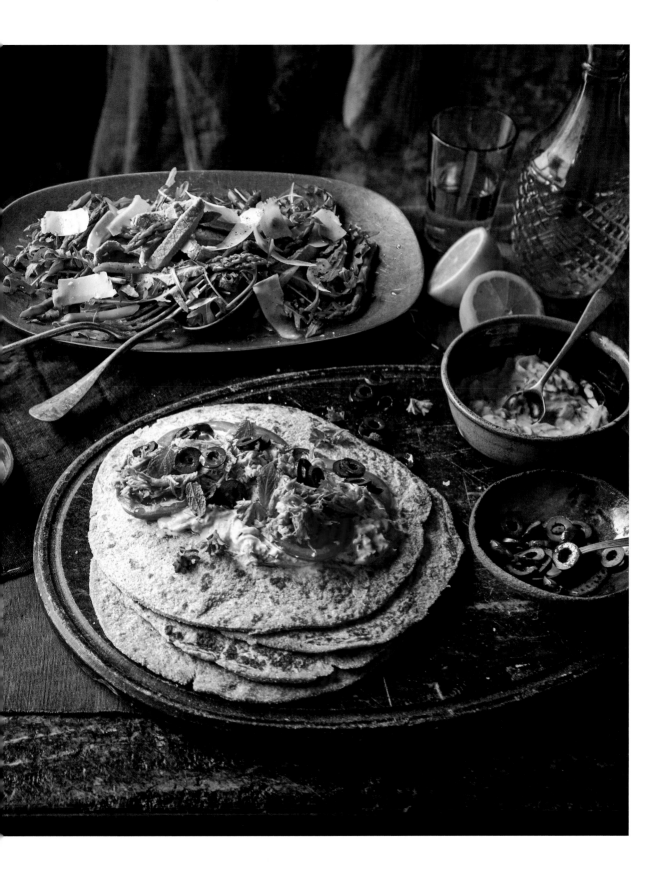

Greek Lamb Wraps

with Tzatziki & Tomatoes

When I roast a leg of lamb, I always enjoy it medium (pink) and sliced. However, when I cook a shoulder, I liked to do so low and slow, meaning the soft flesh can easily be 'pulled' using two forks. Both versions are amazing, and either can be used in the recipe here. Remember though, there may be a lot of fat in lamb, so allow the leftover pieces to gently warm through before using to prevent any chunks of solidified fat. Please note that the times indicated exclude the cooking of the lamb or the making of the wraps. *Pictured on page 35.*

4 SERVINGS

15m PREP TIME

CALORIES 502 | CARBS 9.4G | FAT 30G | PROTEIN 38G

4 Soft Tortilla Wraps (page 72)

1 tomato, thinly sliced

350g (12oz) cooked roast lamb leftovers, sliced or pulled

handful of fresh flat-leaf parsley leaves, finely chopped

small handful of fresh mint leaves

For the tzatziki

200g (7oz) full-fat plain yogurt

140g (5oz) coarsely grated cucumber (drained weight; see Tip)

2 garlic cloves, crushed in a garlic press

very generous handful of fresh mint leaves, finely chopped

squeeze fresh lemon juice, to taste

salt and freshly ground black pepper

For the tzatziki, simply combine all the ingredients together in a small bowl.

Spread the tzatziki on the wraps and add the tomato slices and roast lamb pieces. Generously scatter with equal amounts of chopped parsley and mint leaves and roll up tightly before tucking in!

✳

Why not add some thinly sliced black olives, if you have any to hand?

✳

Place the grated cucumber in a sieve for 5 minutes to drain off excess liquid. This will prevent a watery tzatziki.

OTHER IDEAS FOR USING UP LEFTOVER ROAST LAMB

If you have enough soft-cooked lamb shoulder meat left over, pull it into thinner pieces and use 450g (1lb) in my Cheat's Lasagne (pages 54–5) in place of the Beefy Mince.

SERVES 4 AT 7.1G CARBS PER SERVING

Make Pulled Lamb Sliders using 300g (10½oz) shredded soft-cooked lamb shoulder, with a generous spreading of the tzatziki above on 4 Burger Buns (see page 71).

MAKES 4 AT 6.5G CARBS PER SERVING

Creamy Coconut & Lime Soup

I've never really been one to buy and roast a whole chicken because we tend to always just buy our favourite cut (thighs). But then I realised how affordable – and versatile – a whole bird can be! What follows is what I now do with leftover roast chicken. If you have a larger family, you may as well roast two birds at the same time, enjoying all the juicy cuts for Sunday lunch and the remaining meat (the breasts are ideal) in recipes that call for leftover chicken, like the ones that follow. That's double the pleasure for the same effort. Please note that the time indicated here excludes roasting the chicken or making a homemade stock. *Pictured on page 34.*

CALORIES 367 | CARBS 4.2G | FAT 22G | PROTEIN 37G

4 SERVINGS

10m PREP TIME

25m COOK TIME

1 teaspoon coconut oil

2 garlic cloves, roughly chopped

2 green or red chillies, halved lengthways, plus chilli slices, to garnish

1 teaspoon curry powder

juice of 3 limes

700ml (1¼ pints) chicken stock, see below

small handful of fresh coriander leaves and stalks, plus extra to garnish

400g (14oz) can full-fat coconut milk

400g (14oz) leftover roast chicken, roughly chopped

1 teaspoon powdered erythritol, sifted (optional)

salt and freshly ground black pepper (optional)

Melt the coconut oil in a large non-stick pan or wok over a medium heat. Add the garlic and cook for 1–2 minutes until softened. Add the halved chillies and the curry powder, followed by the lime juice. Cook for 1 minute until all the lime juice evaporates, then pour in the chicken stock. Increase the heat and bring to a strong boil for 8–10 minutes, adding the coriander in the last 30 seconds. Remove from the heat, then strain the infused stock into a large clean pan over a medium heat, discarding the contents of the sieve.

Add the coconut milk to the pan of strained stock (shake the tin well before opening) and whisk well to combine. Now add the cooked chicken pieces and allow the soup to gently reheat for 3–4 minutes. Taste the soup to adjust the seasoning. I like to add a teaspoon of erythritol, along with some salt and pepper.

Divide between 4 bowls and garnish with sliced fresh chillies and/or some finely chopped coriander leaves (optional).

TO MAKE A QUICK HOMEMADE CHICKEN STOCK

After roasting the bird and removing all the meat, remove and discard the contents of the cavity (e.g. any lemon, onion or herbs you may have tucked in there to flavour the chicken). Place the carcass in a medium saucepan. Pour in the fat and juices from the chicken roasting dish, along with 750ml (1⅓ pints) water. Use a wooden spoon to crush the bones so everything is submerged. Bring to the boil, then reduce to a low simmer and cover with a lid to prevent too much evaporation. Cook for 25–30 minutes before straining. I was left with about 700ml (1¼ pints) of delicious chicken stock, which freezes well. It's this lovely, fresh stock that I use in my soup.

Chicken Salad
with Green Goddess Dressing

USING LEFTOVER ROAST CHICKEN

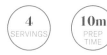

4 SERVINGS **10m** PREP TIME

It's not unusual to use leftover roast chicken in a salad, but here I wanted to showcase this sensational dressing, which includes a generous range of soft herbs and some yogurt. We always have a variety of fresh herbs in the house, because I like to garnish my dishes with them, and this is a great way of using them up. Just so you know, when I refer to 'generous' handfuls, I mean exactly that: don't be shy!

CALORIES 199 | CARBS 2.4G | FAT 4.7G | PROTEIN 36G

150g (5½ oz) full-fat plain yogurt

juice of 1 lemon

generous handful each of fresh chives, roughly chopped, tarragon leaves, flat-leaf parsley leaves, mint leaves and coriander leaves

1 garlic clove, roughly chopped

400g (14oz) leftover roast chicken, roughly chopped

100g (3½oz) salad leaves of your choice

olive oil (optional)

salt and freshly ground black pepper

Place the yogurt, lemon juice (catch the pips!), all the herbs and the garlic in a mini food processor or food chopper. Blitz well until you have a smooth dressing.

Combine the chicken pieces with the dressing and season with salt and freshly ground black pepper. Serve over salad leaves, which you may want to dress with a little olive oil.

If you decide to have this as a packed lunch, keep the chicken mixture and the (undressed) salad leaves in separate containers, then mix together just before eating to prevent wilted leaves.

Chicken
with Red Pepper Cream

USING LEFTOVER ROAST CHICKEN

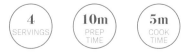

4 SERVINGS **10m** PREP TIME **5m** COOK TIME

Ras el hanout is the delicious dominant flavour here. It combines with leftover roast chicken and jarred roasted red peppers to create a creamy, fragrant chicken 'sauce' that can be served over buttered courgetti or Creamy Cauliflower Rice (page 29). So easy, so lovely!

CALORIES 434 | CARBS 5.6G | FAT 31G | PROTEIN 34G

200g (7oz) jarred roasted red peppers, drained and roughly chopped

200ml (7fl oz) double cream

2 teaspoons unsalted butter

3 garlic cloves, finely chopped

1 tablespoon ras el hanout

400g (14oz) leftover roast chicken, roughly chopped

small handful of fresh mint leaves

salt and freshly ground black pepper

Place the roasted red peppers and cream in a mini food processor and blitz well until you are left with a smooth mixture. Set aside.

Melt the butter in a non-stick frying pan over a medium heat and fry the garlic for 1–2 minutes until softened. Add the ras el hanout and cook for a few more seconds until the pan starts looking dry. Pour in the red pepper cream and continue to cook for 2–3 minutes until the sauce is warmed through and starting to reduce a little. Stir in the cooked chicken pieces to gently warm through and season the mixture with salt and freshly ground black pepper. Serve with a scattering of mint to add a lovely fresh element.

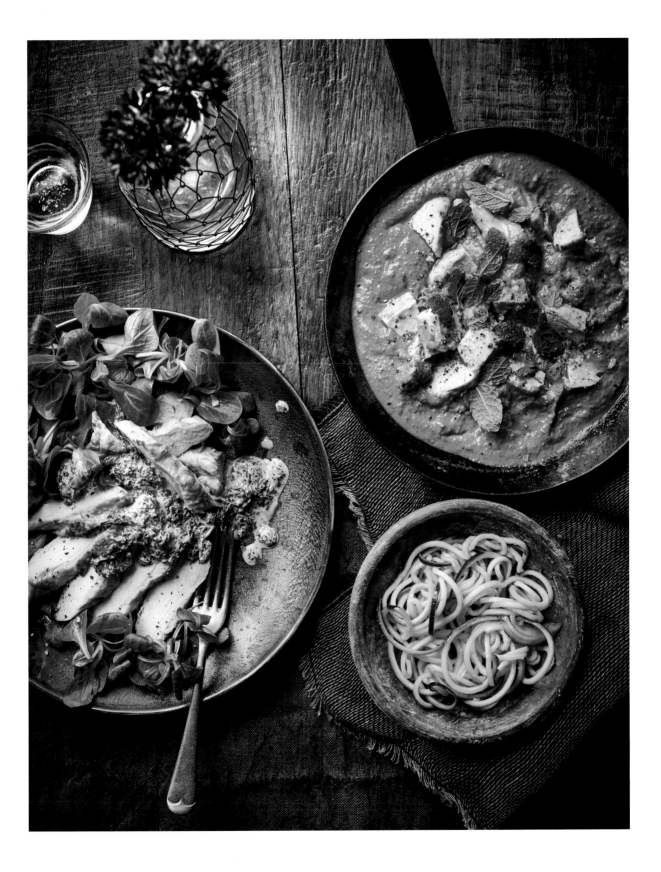

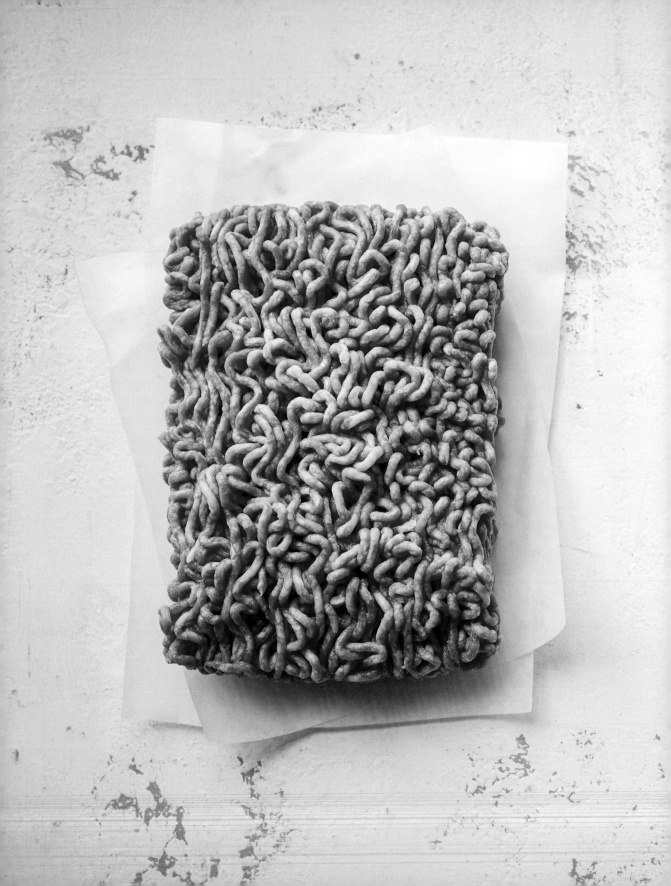

Marvellous Mince

I could quite easily write a whole cookbook called *1000 Ways with Mince*!

I moved out of home soon after I turned 18, and it didn't take me long to realise how inexpensive minced beef was: plus it's easy to cook, and it tastes fabulous. There are so many ways to use it, and it's the base of many crowd-pleasing family favourites, many of which I've shared here.

Luckily for those of us on a keto diet, high-fat mince is lower in price than the leaner kind (at least, it is here in the UK), so I decided to dedicate a whole chapter to ways in which you can enjoy this inexpensive meat as part of a sensational, hearty and comforting meal.

To make things even easier – and more cost-effective – there are many recipes in this chapter that share the same beefy mince mixture as their base, so I decided to include a recipe for a Batch-cooked Beefy Mince (page 42) that can be portioned up and frozen for your convenience, ready to use in your favourite recipes.

And of course, I couldn't forget about meatballs (utterly delicious when spiced and seasoned with love) and good ol' burgers, where I share an interesting topping. There is also a tasty and tempting Cheeseburger Casserole. And it's not just beef: you can try my Mini Pork Sliders, made with minced pork, or try a variation on my Koftas by swapping the minced beef for the more traditionally used lamb (if your budget allows for it).

Mince just got interesting!

Batch-cooked Beefy Mince

This is a super-simple and satisfying beefy mince mixture with myriad uses, as you will see throughout this chapter. Heston Blumenthal recommends adding star anise when frying onions to boost meaty flavours, and he is absolutely right! I like to add red wine to deglaze the pan, but this is optional (although encouraged). Using beef stock not only further tenderises the meat with all that additional simmering, but also adds to the 'beefiness'. This great recipe freezes well after being portioned, but remember that it is not yet seasoned, so check the recipes where it is used because I finish it differently every time. This batch will make enough for three family dinners that serve 4 people.

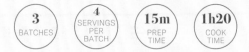

3 BATCHES · **4** SERVINGS PER BATCH · **15m** PREP TIME · **1h20** COOK TIME

PER SERVING (125G): CALORIES 345 | CARBS 1.9G | FAT 27G | PROTEIN 24G

25g (1oz) unsalted butter

1½ onions, finely chopped

3 whole star anise

6 garlic cloves, finely chopped

1.5kg (3lb 5oz) minced beef, 20 per cent fat

180ml (6fl oz) red wine or 3 tablespoons red wine vinegar

500ml (18fl oz) beef stock

FOR A 500G (1LB 2OZ) BATCH

If you haven't pre-made several batches of this Beefy Mince and want to use only a 500g (1lb 2oz) batch in a recipe that calls for it, just make it fresh. Divide the ingredients listed above by 3 (in other words, 2 teaspoons butter, ½ onion, 1 star anise, 2 garlic cloves, 500g/1lb 2oz mince, 60ml/ 2fl oz red wine and 165ml/5½ fl oz stock) and follow the instructions above, then continue with your chosen recipe. Remember, making a smaller batch may mean that the cooking times indicated above will reduce a little.

Melt the butter in your largest non-stick saucepan over a medium heat. Add the onions and star anise and cook for 15–20 minutes until the onions soften and start to caramelise. Add the garlic and continue to cook for 2–3 minutes until the garlic softens, stirring regularly to prevent the garlic burning and turning bitter.

Increase the heat to high and add the mince in a couple of batches, using a wooden spoon to break it up between each addition. Continue to cook, stirring regularly, for 15 minutes until the mince browns evenly and all excess moisture has cooked out. Pour in the wine or red wine vinegar and cook for another 12–15 minutes until the wine completely cooks out and evaporates (you will notice it won't smell as strong), then pour in the beef stock. Bring to the boil, then reduce the heat to medium. Leave to simmer until the beef stock has itself completely evaporated and you are left with only a delicious basic beefy mince mixture. This can take up to 25 minutes. There should be no liquid, apart from fat. Pick out and discard the star anise.

Divide the mixture into three equal-weight batches (approximately 500g/1lb 2oz each) to portion and use in the future for your chosen recipes.

Ultimate Spicy 'Bolognese'

A crowd-pleasing pot of Bolognese will always get your family's vote. I love this with a bit of a kick, so I add chilli powder to the mix and garnish with freshly sliced red chillies – but this is entirely optional. Delicious over courgetti or any of your favourite bases – and don't forget the basil, which (as we know) goes so well with tomatoes and mince! Your cook time will be significantly decreased if you've already prepared a batch of Beefy Mince. *Pictured on page 44.*

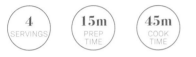

4 SERVINGS | **15m** PREP TIME | **45m** COOK TIME

CALORIES 545 | CARBS 6.7G | FAT 42G | PROTEIN 34G

1 batch (500g/1lb 2oz) pre-cooked Beefy Mince (opposite), defrosted if frozen

400g (14oz) can chopped tomatoes

1 teaspoon unsalted butter

100g (3½oz) smoked streaky bacon, chopped small (see Tip on page 26)

2 teaspoons dried oregano

2 teaspoons chilli powder

2 tablespoon double-concentrated tomato purée

1 tablespoon powdered erythritol, sifted

salt and freshly ground black pepper

To finish

80g (2¾oz) full-fat mature Cheddar cheese, grated

small handful of fresh basil leaves, thinly sliced (see Tip on page 101)

1 large red chilli, sliced (optional)

Either make one batch (500g/1lb 2oz) Beefy Mince according to the instructions on page 42, or if you're using a pre-made batch, heat it up in a large saucepan over a medium heat. Remember, the fat will have solidified when chilled, so make sure you give it enough time to fully warm through.

Meanwhile, blitz the chopped tomatoes in a food processor to form a smooth purée.

Melt the butter in a large non-stick frying pan over a medium heat and cook the bacon for 8–10 minutes until it releases all its juices and just starts to crisp. Add the dried oregano and chilli powder and increase the heat to high. Add this mixture to your cooked beefy mince and stir well to combine, then add the blitzed tomatoes and tomato purée. Bring to a simmer and leave to cook for 25–30 minutes until the mixture reduces to a lovely chunky Bolognese. Stir in the erythritol and taste your mixture, adjusting with salt and pepper.

Serve over buttered courgetti or your favourite low-carb noodles (excluded in the macros) – and don't forget the all-important finishing touches: grated Cheddar, fresh basil and sliced red chilli (if using)!

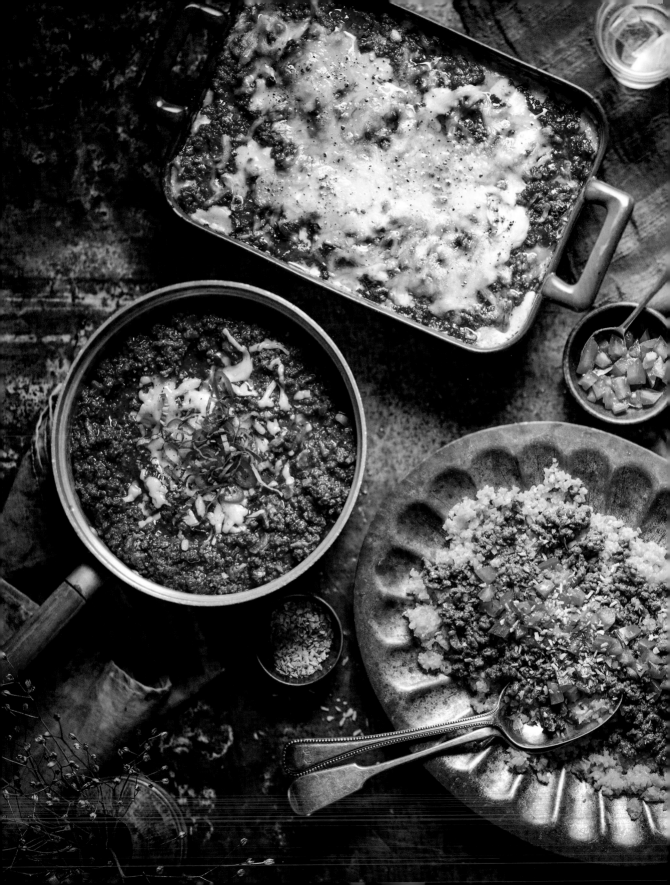

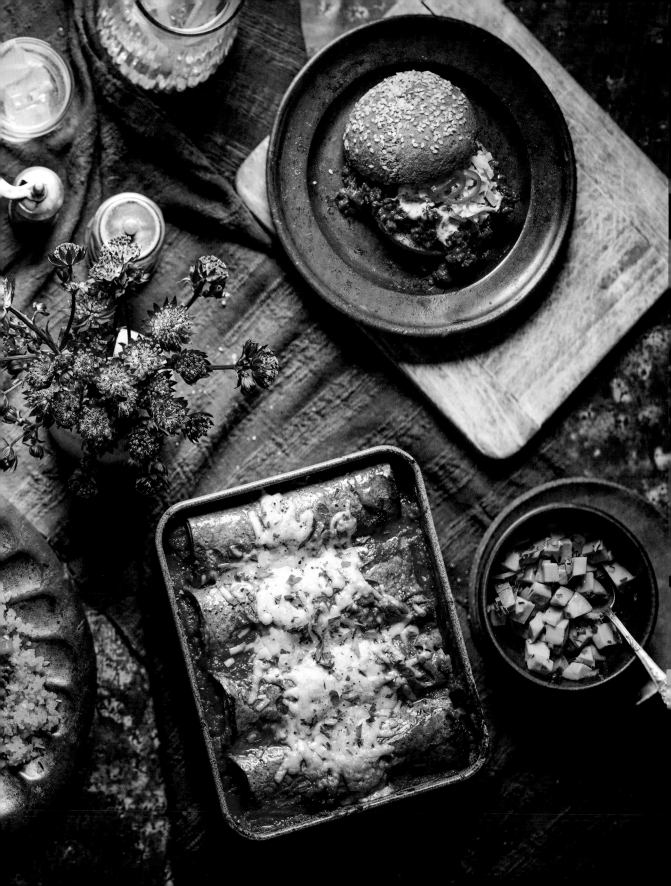

Mum's Curry & Rice

This is a simple, comforting dish that my mum often made us. It's astounding how a handful of simple ingredients could combine to make a meal that I am still thinking about now well into my forties! In South Africa, a traditional 'curry-and-rice' is usually served with sweet elements, like sliced bananas or fruit chutney, so as an alternative, I top mine with chopped tomatoes just before serving to achieve a 'fresh' element – but this is optional. Please note that the times indicated exclude the making of the Curry Butter, and your cook time will be significantly decreased if using pre-cooked Beefy Mince. *Pictured on page 44.*

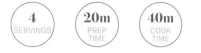

4 SERVINGS   **20m** PREP TIME   **40m** COOK TIME

CALORIES 509 | CARBS 7.7G | FAT 39G | PROTEIN 30G

1 batch (500g/1lb 2oz) pre-cooked Beefy Mince (page 42), defrosted if frozen

1½ tablespoons curry powder

125ml (4fl oz) beef stock

1 teaspoon powdered erythritol, sifted

salt and freshly ground black pepper

For the 'rice'

500g (1lb 2oz) cauliflower florets, blitzed into 'rice' (see page 29 for instructions)

2 teaspoons ground turmeric

4 cardamom pods, lightly crushed with the back of a knife

40g (1½oz) Curry Butter (page 17), approx. 3 slices

To finish

3 tablespoons desiccated coconut

1 tomato, finely chopped (optional)

handful of fresh coriander leaves, finely chopped

Either make one batch (500g/1lb 2oz) Beefy Mince according to the instructions on page 42, or if you're using a pre-made batch, heat it up in a large saucepan over a medium heat. Remember, the fat will have solidified when chilled, so make sure you give it enough time to fully warm through.

Add the curry powder and beef stock to the pan of cooked mince and simmer over a medium heat for 15–20 minutes until the mixture reduces to a lovely thick and chunky consistency. Stir in the erythritol and taste, adjusting with salt and pepper as needed.

Meanwhile, prepare your 'rice'. Bring a large pan of salted water to the boil and add the cauliflower 'rice', turmeric and crushed cardamom pods. Boil rapidly for 3–4 minutes before draining well in a large sieve. Stir in the Curry Butter (see Tip) and allow to melt into the cauliflower. Pick out and discard the cardamom pods, then season with salt and pepper and set aside to keep warm until your mince is ready.

When you're almost ready to serve, toast the desiccated coconut in a hot, dry pan over a medium heat for 3–4 minutes until golden brown. Stir regularly and keep your eye on it – it can quickly burn.

Serve the warm 'rice' with the curried mince and top with the chopped tomato (if using), toasted coconut and chopped coriander.

✳

If you prefer not to use the Curry Butter, simply use regular butter, but add a little more curry powder to your mince mixture.

Spicy Beef Enchiladas

Enchiladas! Well, my version, at least, made with the 'lasagne sheets' featured in my Cheat's Lasagne – they are easier to make than you think! I have not included the cooking time for these here, but they can be made ahead and kept in the fridge. Your cooking time will also be significantly decreased if using pre-cooked Beefy Mince. The optional avocado and red onion salsa complements the enchiladas perfectly, and while it is not included in the macros, it's a beautiful, acidic addition that rounds off every mouthful. *Pictured on page 45.*

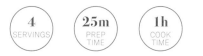

4 SERVINGS | **25m** PREP TIME | **1h** COOK TIME

CALORIES 726 | CARBS 9.6G | FAT 56G | PROTEIN 42G

1 batch (500g/1lb 2oz) pre-cooked Beefy Mince (page 42), defrosted if frozen

1 teaspoon ground cumin

½ teaspoon chilli powder

1 quantity Lasagne Sheets (page 54), sliced into 4 equal-sized wraps

30g (1oz) Parmesan or Pecorino cheese, finely grated

60g (2¼oz) full-fat mature Cheddar cheese, finely grated

handful of fresh parsley leaves, finely chopped

salt flakes, salt and freshly ground black pepper

For the sauce

400g (14oz) can chopped tomatoes

1 tablespoon double-concentrated tomato purée

1 teaspoon ground cumin

½ teaspoon chilli powder

½ teaspoon dried oregano

1 teaspoon powdered erythritol (optional)

For the avocado salsa (optional)

2 avocados, roughly chopped

½ small red onion, very finely chopped

generous squeeze of fresh lemon juice

handful of fresh coriander leaves, finely chopped

Either make one batch (500g/1lb 2oz) Beefy Mince according to the instructions on page 42, or if you're using a pre-made batch, heat it up in a large saucepan over a medium heat. Remember, the fat will have solidified when chilled, so give it enough time to fully warm through. Add the cumin and chilli powder to the cooked mince and cook for 2–3 minutes, stirring well. Set aside for now.

Combine all the sauce ingredients in a small pan over a medium heat. Cook for 10–12 minutes until the tomatoes break down. Take off the heat and use a hand blender to blitz until smooth. Add 3 tablespoons of this mixture to the pan of cooked mince and stir to combine.

Taste both the mince mixture and the tomato sauce and adjust the seasoning with salt and freshly ground black pepper. If you feel the tomato mixture needs it, add the erythritol.

Preheat the oven to 200°C/180°C fan/400°F/gas mark 6.

Spread a little of the tomato sauce on the bottom of a baking dish (which should be the right size for the 4 rolled enchiladas to fit snugly together). Divide the mince mixture between your 4 wraps, placing it on the bottom half of each one, and scatter over a little grated Parmesan. Gently roll up each wrap. Place in the dish, then spoon the remaining tomato sauce around the wraps. Scatter over the grated Cheddar and cover loosely with foil. Bake for 20–25 minutes, removing the foil for the last 4–5 minutes.

If you choose to make the avocado salsa, simply combine all the ingredients and leave covered in the fridge until needed.

Serve the enchiladas garnished generously with finely chopped parsley, with the avocado salsa alongside, if using.

Stuffed Savoy Parcels

Get creative with mince and Savoy cabbage and spend some time making these attractive little parcels! I love the toasted pine nuts, but if they are a little over your budget, try any other toasted nut – they will still add a lovely texture and flavour. If you have nut allergies, though, these parcels are equally delicious without. Your cooking time will be significantly decreased if using pre-cooked Beefy Mince (page 42). Macros are calculated per parcel, but if your daily macros allow for it, you will probably want to tuck into two!

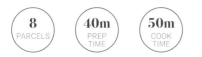

8 PARCELS   **40m** PREP TIME   **50m** COOK TIME

CALORIES 289 | CARBS 6.3 | FAT 22 | PROTEIN 17G

1 batch (500g/1lb 2oz) pre-cooked Beefy Mince (page 42), defrosted if frozen

2 tablespoons unsalted butter

200g (7oz) mushrooms, finely chopped

30g (1oz) pine nuts, toasted and roughly chopped

8 large Savoy cabbage leaves

100g (3½oz) fresh mozzarella, torn into smaller pieces

salt, salt flakes and freshly ground black pepper

For the sauce

400g (14oz) can chopped tomatoes

1 tablespoon double-concentrated tomato purée

2 teaspoons dried oregano

handful of fresh basil leaves, thinly sliced (see Tip on page 101)

1 teaspoon powdered erythritol, sifted (optional)

Preheat the oven to 200°C/180°C/400°F/ gas mark 6.

Either make one batch (500g/1lb 2oz) Beefy Mince according to the instructions on page 42, or if you're using a pre-made batch, heat it up in a large saucepan over a medium heat. Remember, the fat will have solidified when chilled, so give it enough time to fully warm through.

In a large frying pan, melt the butter over a medium–high heat. Add the mushrooms and cook for 5–6 minutes until caramelised, then transfer them to the saucepan with the mince, along with most of the chopped pine nuts.

For the sauce, blitz the chopped tomatoes to a smooth purée in a mini food processor, then add to a small non-stick pan, along with the tomato purée and dried oregano. Cook over a medium heat for 10–11 minutes until it reduces and thickens. Stir in most of the sliced basil, then spoon about a quarter of this sauce into the mince mixture, mixing well to combine. Season to taste, stirring in erythritol if needed.

Bring a large pan of salted water to the boil. Working in two or three batches, boil the cabbage leaves for about 3 minutes until wilted and pliable. Drain on a tray lined with paper towels.

Pour half the sauce into a roasting dish. Cut out a triangle about 2.5cm (1in) long from the hard centre of each cabbage leaf, then divide the mince between the 8 leaves and fold into little parcels. Place in the roasting dish, folded side down. Spoon the remaining tomato sauce in between the parcels, then scatter the mozzarella over the top. Cover with foil (pierced a few times with a fork) and bake for 25 minutes.

Season, then scatter over the remaining basil and pine nuts to serve.

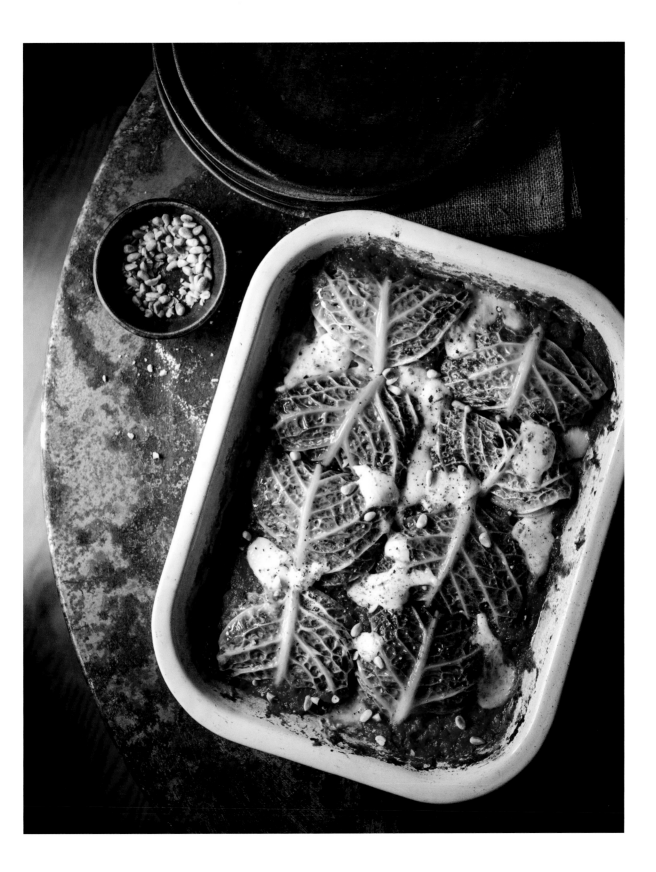

Smoky Sloppy Joes

Messy – but fun! Mark and I love 'Sloppy Joe Nights', and we tuck in like two kids eating with abandon! If you prefer to eat these with a little more class, you could spoon the smoky mince on to two halves and enjoy this with cutlery – but, where's the fun in that?! The smoked paprika here offers that distinct smoky flavour that takes these to the next level. Please note that the prep time doesn't include the making of the buns, but they are included in the macros. Your cooking time will be significantly decreased if using pre-cooked Beefy Mince (page 42). *Pictured on page 45.*

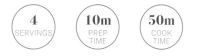

4 SERVINGS | **10m** PREP TIME | **50m** COOK TIME

CALORIES 726 | CARBS 9.8G | FAT 58G | PROTEIN 41G

1 batch (500g/1lb 2oz) pre-cooked Beefy Mince (page 42), defrosted if frozen

1 teaspoon smoked paprika

1 teaspoon chilli powder

400g (14oz) can chopped tomatoes

250ml (9fl oz) beef stock

4 Burger Buns (page 71)

4 tablespoons soured cream

60g (2¼oz) full-fat mature Cheddar cheese, grated

1 red chilli, finely sliced (optional)

salt and freshly ground black pepper

Either make one batch (500g/1lb 2oz) Beefy Mince according to the instructions on page 42, or if you're using a pre-made batch, heat it up in a large saucepan over a medium heat. Remember, the fat will have solidified when chilled, so make sure you give it enough time to fully warm through.

Add the smoked paprika and chilli powder to the pan of cooked mince and stir well to combine, then add the chopped tomatoes and beef stock and bring to the boil. Reduce the heat to low and simmer, uncovered, for 40–45 minutes, stirring occasionally, until you have a thick, chunky mixture. Season with salt and freshly ground black pepper.

Halve the buns (which are best enjoyed warm) and divide the mixture between the bottom halves. Top with the soured cream, grated cheese and sliced red chillies (if using) before covering each bun with its top half.

✳

This is a very satisfying dish after a day of fasting. However, if you find the carbs too high, make a 'half-Sloppy' and enjoy half a dressed bun with a salad instead.

Nacho Beef Bowl

with Soured Cream Guacamole

What a fabulous dish for the family to indulge in while playing board games! This recipe is not as complicated as you may think, because many elements can be made ahead of time. The nachos take a while, but they can be made earlier in the day (or even the day before) – and I have offered ways to bring them back to life if they lose their 'crispness'. The macros are for 4 people, but if you find the carbs too high for this recipe, serve this as part of an appetiser spread for a party of 6–8 people, and get creative with your platter! More chopped tomatoes and chillies are always welcome! *Pictured on page 52.*

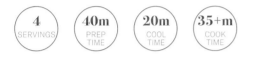

4 SERVINGS | **40m** PREP TIME | **20m** COOL TIME | **35+m** COOK TIME

CALORIES 606 | CARBS 11G | FAT 44G | PROTEIN 36G

1 batch (500g/1lb 2oz) pre-cooked Beefy Mince (page 42), defrosted if frozen

½ tablespoon chilli powder

2 tomatoes, finely chopped

1 tablespoon double-concentrated tomato purée

30g (1oz) jalapeños in brine, drained and finely chopped

200ml (7fl oz) water

50g (1¾oz) full-fat mature Cheddar cheese, grated

salt and freshly ground black pepper

1–2 red or green chillies, finely sliced, to serve (optional)

For the nachos

2 large eggs, whisked

30g (1oz) nutritional yeast flakes

2 tablespoons arrowroot powder (or use 2 x 8g/¼oz sachets)

1 teaspoon garlic powder

1 teaspoon salt

1 tablespoon psyllium husk powder

(ingredients continued overleaf)

Begin with the nachos, as they can be made ahead of time. Preheat the oven to 200°C/180°C fan/400°F/gas mark 6, and get out 2 large baking trays, a large silicone mat and a large sheet of baking paper.

Place the whisked eggs, yeast flakes, arrowroot powder, garlic powder and salt in a bowl. Use a hand blender to mix them together very well, ensuring there are no lumps. Whisk in the psyllium husk powder.

You will be left with a fairly pourable mixture, but the psyllium will thicken it over time, so it's best to tip the mixture out on to your silicone mat as soon as it's well mixed. Use a spoon or small spatula to spread out the mixture to create a thin, large rectangle, about 25 x 30cm (10 x 12in). Make sure the mixture is spread thinly, evenly and without visible holes. Slide the silicone mat on to one of the baking trays and bake on the lowest rack in the oven for 6 minutes.

Remove from the oven and place the sheet of baking paper on top of the partially baked mixture, then place the second baking tray upside down on top of it. Carefully flip the whole lot over. Your partially baked mixture will now be on the second tray, with the baking paper underneath it. Slowly peel off the silicone mat.

Use a pizza cutter to slice the partially baked mixture into 15 squares, then halve each diagonally to create triangles. Separate the triangles slightly and switch the outer and inner pieces to ensure even baking.

Return the tray to the oven for another 8–9 minutes, switching some nachos around if you feel they are darkening too much. Once they have all cooked beautifully, remove from the oven and transfer the nachos from the tray to a wire rack for 20 minutes.

✻ *continued overleaf*

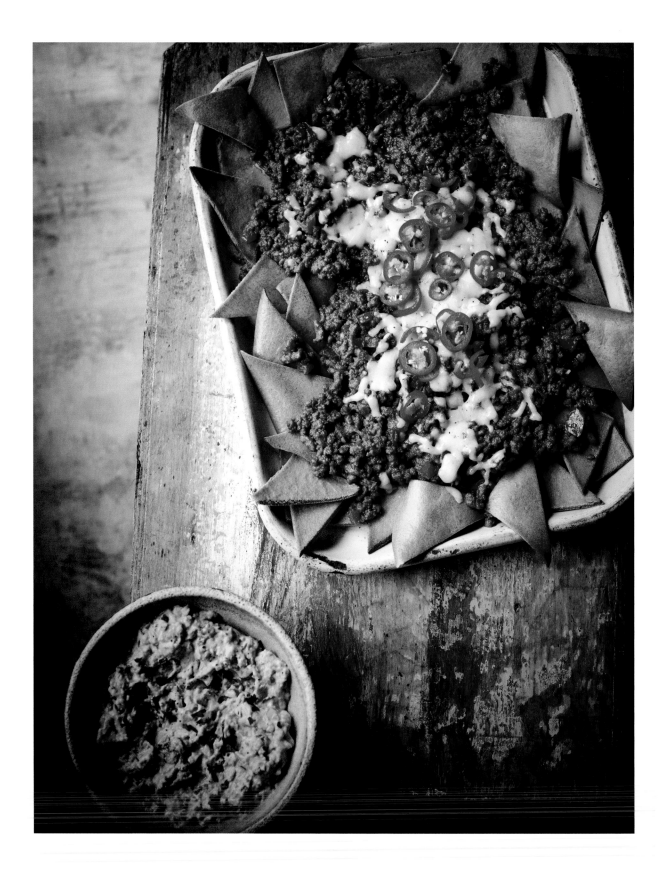

Nacho
Beef Bowl

with Soured Cream Guacamole (continued)

For the soured cream guacamole

1 avocado, roughly chopped

40g (1½oz) soured cream

juice of ½ lime

small handful of fresh coriander leaves, finely chopped

¼ red onion, very finely chopped

*

I add the chopped fresh tomatoes in two stages so that some of them cook down and add to the overall flavour, and some bring a lovely freshness.

If, after 20 minutes, the nachos are not crisp enough, place the rack containing the nachos over a baking tray and place in the oven (on its lowest setting) for 15–20 minutes. This should crisp them up further without burning them. (Alternatively, you could pop them in an air-fryer on the dehydrator setting.)

Moving on! Either make one batch (500g/1lb 2oz) Beefy Mince according to the instructions on page 42, or if you're using a pre-made batch, heat it up in a large saucepan over a medium heat. Remember, the fat will have solidified when chilled, so make sure you give it enough time to fully warm through.

Add the chilli powder to the pan and stir well to combine, then add half the chopped tomatoes, along with the tomato purée, chopped jalapeños and water. Simmer for 14–15 minutes until the mixture is lovely and chunky, and free of excess liquid. Add the remaining chopped tomatoes (see Tip) and cook for another minute before seasoning with salt and pepper. Set aside to keep warm.

For the soured cream guacamole, mash the avocado with the soured cream and lime juice using the back of a fork. (Alternatively, blitz in a mini food processor or food chopper for a smoother mixture.) Season with salt and pepper and stir in the chopped coriander and red onion. (The red onion adds small, sweet crunchy bits, so be sure it is diced very small to avoid overpowering the flavour of the guacamole.)

Top the nachos with the spicy beef and scatter the Cheddar over the beef so it melts. Scatter over the chillies, if using, then serve with the soured cream guacamole alongside.

Cheat's Lasagne

This comforting 'lasagne' will serve anything between 4 and 6 people (depending on how hungry they are!): I based the macros on a 250g (9oz) cooked serving to help you make the best choice when portioning. For this dish, I've created a faux lasagne layer using a combination of mascarpone cheese and psyllium husk powder. It may not be the real thing, but it adds a textured layer and does a far better job of soaking up flavours than courgettes or aubergines, which are often used in keto lasagnes. As ever, your cook time will be significantly decreased if using pre-cooked Beefy Mince. *Pictured on page 44.*

CALORIES 731 | CARBS 8.5G | FAT 63G | PROTEIN 31G

4-6 SERVINGS | **30m** PREP TIME | **45m** COOK TIME

1 batch (500g/1lb 2oz) pre-cooked Beefy Mince (page 42), defrosted if frozen

400g (14oz) can chopped tomatoes

2 tablespoons double-concentrated tomato purée

small handful of fresh basil leaves, finely sliced

salt and freshly ground black pepper

For the 'lasagne' sheets

4 large eggs

150g (5½oz) mascarpone

1 teaspoon garlic powder

25g (1oz) psyllium husk powder

For the cheesy white sauce

200ml (7fl oz) double cream

150g (5½oz) soured cream

2 tablespoons finely grated Parmesan or Pecorino cheese

generous pinch of ground nutmeg

ground white pepper

Preheat the oven to 180°C/160°C fan/350°F/gas mark 4 and line a very large baking tray with a silicone mat. Have a large sheet of baking paper on hand.

To make the 'lasagne' sheets, place the eggs, mascarpone, garlic powder and a very generous pinch of salt in a large bowl. Use a hand blender to blitz the mixture until smooth and free of lumps. Add the psyllium husk powder and blitz well to combine. The psyllium husk powder will soon stiffen the mixture, so pour it out on to the lined tray and cover with the sheet of baking paper. Use your hands over the top of the baking paper to spread out the mixture into a large, thin sheet. My lasagne dish is 29 x 18cm (11½ x 7in), so to make two layers, I made sure the mixture was spread out to 29 x 36cm (11½ x 14in).

Bake on the lowest rack in the oven for 5 minutes, then reduce the temperature to 160°C/140°C fan/325°F/gas mark 3 and bake for another 10–11 minutes. Carefully peel away the top layer of baking paper, gently nudging any small areas that may have stuck. Don't be alarmed if it has risen in places: this is because of the eggs, and it will settle! Slice into 2 equal-sized pieces to make your layers. Set aside.

Next, either make one batch (500g/1lb 2oz) Beefy Mince according to the instructions on page 42, or if you're using a pre-made batch, heat it up in a large saucepan over a medium heat. Remember, the fat will have solidified when chilled, so make sure you give it enough time to fully warm through.

To finish

70g (2½oz) mozzarella (or Cheddar, whatever you have on hand), grated

1 tablespoon finely grated Parmesan or Pecorino cheese

*

These faux 'lasagne' sheets are easier to make than you think, so please give them a try. I also use them as the 'wraps' in my Spicy Beef Enchiladas (page 47).

Add the chopped tomatoes and tomato purée to the pan of cooked mince. Reduce the heat to low and leave to simmer for 25–30 minutes until all excess moisture is cooked out and you are left with a thick, chunky mixture. Taste and adjust the seasoning with salt and pepper. Stir through the sliced basil and set aside until needed.

Meanwhile, make the white sauce. Combine the cream, soured cream and Parmesan in a small pan over a low–medium heat. Season with ground nutmeg, salt and ground white pepper and stir regularly as the cream reduces and thickens a little. This will take about 5–6 minutes.

Now that all your elements are made, it's time to layer up the dish! Increase the oven temperature to 200°C/180°C fan/400°F/gas mark 6.

Spread a very thin layer of the mince mixture on the bottom of your lasagne dish. Cover with one of your 'lasagne' sheets, then top with a generous drizzle of the white sauce, spreading it out evenly with a silicone spatula. Cover this with half the remaining mince mixture, then repeat the process with the remaining 'lasagne' sheet, and some more white sauce. Top with the remaining mince and, if there is any more white sauce, drizzle this over the top. Scatter over the mozzarella and Parmesan, then bake for 20–25 minutes until the whole lot has warmed through and the cheese on top has turned golden. Serve!

Cheeseburger Casserole
with Tomato Burger Sauce

Sometimes I want the taste of a rich, beefy burger without an accompanying low-carb bun (which can often seem quite 'heavy'). I've also never been one to wrap a dressed burger patty in a lettuce leaf! I would rather pick up a knife and fork (gasp!) and enjoy the flavours and classic accompaniments in this tasty casserole. The best part is the chunky burger sauce: I stirred in diced tomatoes, and the freshness it brings is unbeatable! Quick tip: check the labels of gherkins and cornichons. Some contain more sugar than others, so select the ones lowest in carbs.

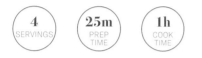

4 SERVINGS **25m** PREP TIME **1h** COOK TIME

CALORIES 762 | CARBS 5.4G | FAT 62G | PROTEIN 44G

2 teaspoons unsalted butter

100g (3½oz) smoked bacon lardons (or smoked streaky bacon, finely chopped)

½ onion, finely chopped

2 garlic cloves, finely chopped

500g (1lb 2oz) minced beef, 20 per cent fat

40g (1½oz) full-fat cream cheese

25g (1oz) gherkins or cornichons, finely chopped

salt and freshly ground black pepper

For the cheese layer

1 large egg

100g (3½oz) full-fat cream cheese

2 teaspoons American-style mustard

100g (3½oz) full-fat mature Cheddar cheese, finely grated

25g (1oz) gherkins or cornichons, finely chopped

For the tomato burger sauce

1 tomato, finely chopped

50g (1¾oz) mayonnaise

50g (1¾oz) no-added-sugar ketchup

Preheat the oven to 200°C/180°C fan/400°F/gas mark 6.

Melt half the butter in a large non-stick pan over a medium heat. Add the bacon lardons and cook for 8–10 minutes until they release all their moisture and are cooked through. Remove using a slotted spoon (leaving all the juice and fat in the pan) and set aside on a plate.

Add the remaining butter to the pan with the bacon juices and cook the onion for 9–10 minutes until it starts to soften. Add the garlic and cook for another 1–2 minutes until the onion starts to caramelise and the garlic softens. Add the mince and increase the heat to high. Break up the mince, stirring regularly for 6–7 minutes until evenly browned. Remove from the heat and stir in the cream cheese, gherkins and cooked bacon. Adjust the seasoning with plenty of pepper (see Tip).

Transfer the mixture to an ovenproof dish (approximately 18 x 18 cm/7 x 7in) and press the mince down, making sure there's space to add the cheese layer later. Cover with foil and make several little holes with a toothpick. Bake for 20 minutes.

To prepare the cheese layer, whisk together the egg, cream cheese and mustard in a bowl. Stir in the grated cheese and gherkins.

Once the burger layer has been baking for 20 minutes, remove the tray from the oven and discard the foil. If you notice a lot of excess grease on the top, blot with paper towels. Pour the creamy cheese mixture over the top of the meat, then return to the oven for 15 minutes.

Mix together the tomato burger sauce ingredients in a small bowl.

Slice the casserole into 4 equal portions and serve with a lovely dollop of the chunky burger sauce.

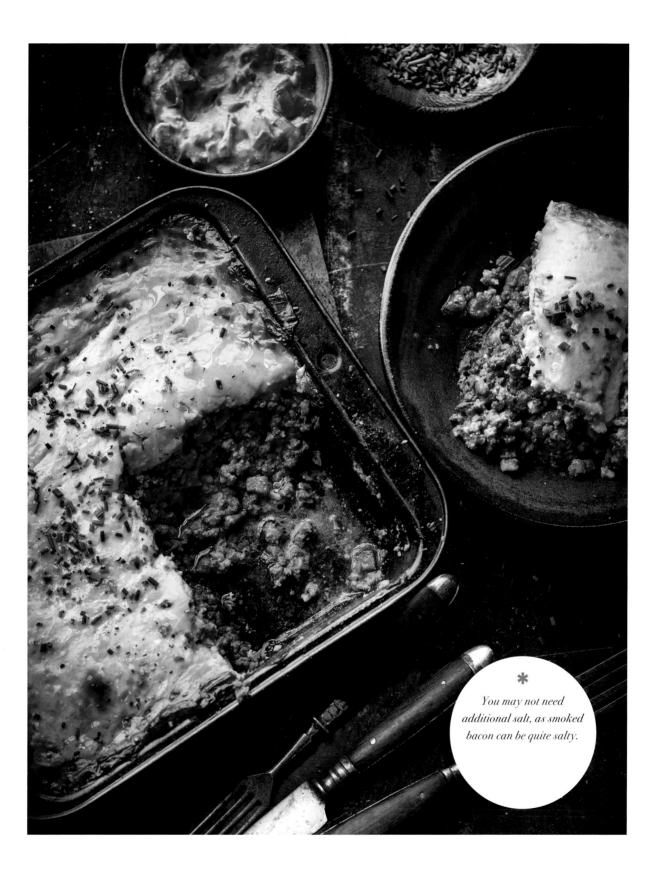

*

You may not need
additional salt, as smoked
bacon can be quite salty.

Fragrant Meatballs

with Herby 'Couscous'

This book will be worth your moolah just for this dynamite recipe alone! A bold statement, I realise, but there are incredible flavours that can be achieved from some minced beef, a few spices from your pantry and some leftover herbs. This is a truly special meal – and happens to be quite similar to one I make for my favourite athlete when I do my regular private-cheffing gig over the Wimbledon Championship every year. I hope you love it as much as my client does: it's just beautiful! *Pictured here with Baharat Meatballs with Courgette & Minty Feta Salad (see page 60).*

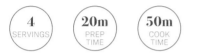

4 SERVINGS   **20m** PREP TIME   **50m** COOK TIME

CALORIES 494 | CARBS 7.3G | FAT 38G | PROTEIN 29G

500g (1lb 2oz) minced beef, 20 per cent fat

2 teaspoons ground cumin

½ teaspoon chilli powder

¼ teaspoons ground cinnamon

¼ teaspoons garlic powder

pinch of ground allspice

1 tablespoon ghee or lard

salt and freshly ground black pepper

For the cauliflower 'couscous'

55g (2oz) unsalted butter

550g (1lb 4oz) cauliflower florets, blitzed into 'rice' (see page 29 for instructions)

½ teaspoon dried oregano

½ onion, finely chopped

3 garlic cloves, finely chopped

1 teaspoon ground cumin

generous handful of fresh flat-leaf parsley leaves, finely chopped

generous handful of fresh coriander leaves, finely chopped

small handful of fresh mint leaves, finely chopped

small handful of fresh dill, finely chopped

1 tomato, finely chopped

juice of ½ lemon

Preheat the oven to 200°C/180°C fan/400°F/gas mark 6 and line a large baking tray with baking paper.

Begin by preparing the cauliflower. Melt the butter in a small pan over a medium heat. Once melted, pour it into the bowl of blitzed cauliflower 'rice'. Mix well, then tip out on to the lined tray and spread out evenly. Bake for 20–25 minutes, stirring every 10 minutes. Transfer to a bowl and stir through the oregano. Set aside, and reduce the oven temperature to 150°C/130°C fan/300°F/gas mark 2.

In a large bowl, combine the mince with the cumin, chilli powder, cinnamon, garlic powder and allspice. Season generously with salt and pepper and form the mixture into 12 meatballs (see Tip on page 63).

Melt the ghee or lard in a large non-stick pan over a high heat and brown the meatballs for 1–2 minutes until golden and caramelised on the outside. Do this in a couple of batches to avoid overcrowding your pan. Remove using a slotted spoon (leaving the juices in the pan) and place on a small baking tray. Transfer to the oven for 15–17 minutes to gently finish cooking through.

Meanwhile, to finish the cauliflower, place the same pan you used for the meatballs over a medium heat. Add the onion and cook in the pan's juices for about 8–10 minutes until softened and starting to caramelise. Add the garlic and cumin and cook for another minute. Tip in the cauliflower mixture and stir everything together. Once warm, remove the pan from the heat and stir in all the chopped herbs, as well as the tomato and lemon juice (catch the pips!). Stir well to combine.

By now, the meatballs should have finished cooking through. Serve them over the herby 'couscous' and season with salt and pepper.

*

If any juices ran from the
meatballs while they were
in the oven, drizzle this over
the cauliflower couscous for
maximum flavour!

Baharat Meatballs

with Courgette & Minty Feta Salad

This is a delicious warm salad you can enjoy in the summer months, and I love it because we so often associate mince with winter cooking. These beautifully spiced, fragrant meatballs are served over sliced courgettes (chargrilled for maximum flavour), then finished with a dash of acidic balsamic and a crumbling of salty feta. And the mint leaves: please don't skip them, they are sensational as a fresh garnish here. *Pictured on page 59.*

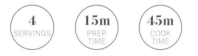

4 SERVINGS | **15m** PREP TIME | **45m** COOK TIME

CALORIES 648 | CARBS 6.5G | FAT 53G | PROTEIN 34G

1 tablespoon unsalted butter

1 onion, finely chopped

2 garlic cloves, finely chopped

1 teaspoon apple cider vinegar

500g (1lb 2oz) minced beef, 20 per cent fat

2 tablespoons baharat spice mix

1 tablespoon ghee or lard

salt and freshly ground black pepper

For the courgette salad

180g (6½oz) full-fat feta cheese

very generous handful of fresh mint leaves, finely chopped

3 tablespoons olive oil

3 tablespoons unflavoured (odourless) coconut oil or ghee

600g (1lb 5oz) courgettes, sliced at an angle into 1cm (½in) slices (trimmed weight)

1 teaspoon balsamic vinegar

Preheat the oven to 150°C/130°C fan/300°F/gas mark 2.

Melt the butter in a small frying pan over a low–medium heat. Add the onion and cook for 18–20 minutes until it completely softens and starts to caramelise, but don't let it burn. Add the garlic and continue to cook for 1–2 minutes until the garlic softens, then add the apple cider vinegar. Cook for another minute, or until there is no moisture present in the pan. Remove from the heat.

Tip the mince into a large bowl and scatter over the baharat spice mix. Add the caramelised onion mixture and season with salt and pepper. Stir to combine, then form 24 even-sized little meatballs from the mixture (see Tip on page 63).

Melt the lard or ghee in a large non-stick pan over a high heat and fry the meatballs for 1–2 minutes until browned on the outside. Do this in two batches to avoid overcrowding your pan. Transfer to a baking tray and place in the oven to finish cooking through for 14–15 minutes.

Meanwhile, to make the salad, crumble the feta in a bowl and stir through the chopped mint. Drizzle over the olive oil and season with freshly ground black pepper. Set aside.

Melt the coconut oil or ghee in a griddle pan over a high heat. Fry the sliced courgettes, working in 3–4 batches, for about 1 minute on each side or until you see visible char marks. Remove and place on a tray lined with paper towels to drain, then transfer to a bowl and drizzle over the balsamic vinegar. Season with salt and toss to combine.

Serve the meatballs over the griddled courgettes, then spoon the marinated minty feta over the top.

Koftas in Warm 'Pita'

with Tzatziki & Tomatoes

This is a whopper of a recipe, but it's because I want you to achieve the best results, so I tried to give as much detail as possible. You will love the warm 'pita', which is loosely based on my soft tortilla recipe (page 72), with a few minor adjustments. Koftas are popularly made with lamb mince, but I used the more affordable, easily available beef mince – and, if seasoned well, it's unlikely you will notice much of a difference. With this recipe, each person will enjoy two prepared koftas with all the trimmings! *Pictured on page 62.*

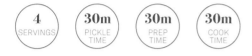

| 4 SERVINGS | 30m PICKLE TIME | 30m PREP TIME | 30m COOK TIME |

CALORIES 739 | CARBS 11G | FAT 57G | PROTEIN 35G

500g (1lb 2oz) minced beef, 20 per cent fat (or minced lamb, if you prefer)

1 teaspoon ground cumin

1 teaspoon ground coriander

1 teaspoon garlic powder

1 teaspoon dried oregano

2 tablespoons lard or ghee

salt, salt flakes and freshly ground pepper

1 quantity Tzatziki (page 36), to serve

For the 'pita' breads

325g (11½oz) warm water

1 teaspoon inulin powder

10g (¼oz) dried active yeast

110g (3¾oz) coconut flour

3 tablespoons psyllium husk powder

½ teaspoon dried oregano

½ teaspoon salt

2 tablespoons olive oil

4 teaspoons lard or ghee (see Tip overleaf)

(ingredients continued overleaf)

Start by prepping the salad. Place the red onion in a small bowl and pour over the cider vinegar. Cover and leave to 'pickle' at room temperature for at least 30 minutes. Lay the tomato slices out on a large plate and sprinkle over the dried oregano. Drizzle over the olive oil and crack over some black pepper. Cover and leave at room temperature until needed.

Make the 'pita' breads next. Pour the warm water into bowl. Stir in the inulin powder to dissolve. Leave the water to cool until tepid (hot water will kill the yeast), then scatter the yeast over the top and stir well to combine. Set aside for 15 minutes until the surface is frothy and the mixture has grown significantly in size.

In a second, large bowl, combine the coconut flour, psyllium husk powder, dried oregano and salt.

Whisk the olive oil into the yeast mixture until emulsified, then pour the yeast mixture into the coconut flour mixture and stir to combine (work quickly, as the psyllium husk powder will stiffen the mixture rapidly). Smooth over the mixture, pressing it down. Cover the surface directly with clingfilm to prevent the dough from drying out and leave to sit for 2 minutes.

Next, divide the dough into 8 equal-sized portions – they should be about 60g (2¼oz) each. Roll each one into a ball, then place on a large silicone mat. Use your hands to flatten each ball into an oval shape, about 13 x 10cm (5 x 4in). Use your fingers to smooth the perimeter in case the outer edges 'crack' after flattening. Keep the remaining portions covered at all times to prevent drying out.

✱ *continued overleaf*

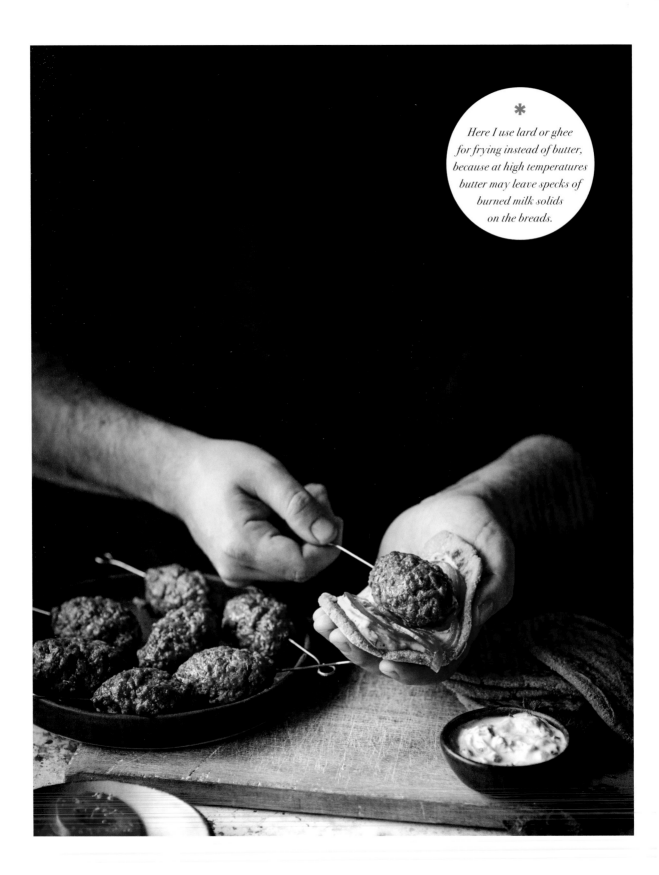

*

*Here I use lard or ghee
for frying instead of butter,
because at high temperatures
butter may leave specks of
burned milk solids
on the breads.*

Koftas in Warm 'Pita'

with Tzatziki & Tomatoes (continued)

For the salad

¼ red onion, very thinly sliced

1 tablespoon apple cider vinegar

1 large tomato, thinly sliced

pinch of dried oregano

2 tablespoons olive oil

*

A bit of quick maths will help you make even-sized meatballs. Weigh your seasoned mince, then divide by the number of meatballs required. Weigh your first one so that you can visually gauge the size you're after.

Heat no more than 1 teaspoon ghee in a large, non-stick pan over a medium–high heat and wipe the melted ghee around the pan with a paper towel. Cook the 'pitas' for 1 minute–1 minute 30 seconds per side, cooking two at a time and using a spatula to flip them. Set aside to keep warm on a plate lined with paper towels and repeat until all of the 'pitas' are cooked. These are best enjoyed warm, so if you make them ahead of time, keep them in the fridge and reheat in a warm oven (120°C/100°C fan/250°F/gas mark ½) for 10–15 minutes. They won't open like pockets as traditional pitas do, but they still do the job!

To make the koftas, preheat the oven to 140°C/120°C fan/275°F/gas mark 1 and line a baking sheet with baking paper. Combine the mince, cumin, coriander, garlic powder and dried oregano in a large bowl. Season very generously with salt and pepper. Divide the mixture into 8 equal-sized portions (see Tip) and form into very compact balls, then shape further into longer little logs. Insert a short skewer into each one lengthways and set aside.

Melt half the lard or ghee in a large non-stick pan over a high heat. Working in batches (and adding the remaining fat halfway through, if needed), gently brown the outside of each kofta for 1–2 minutes, turning to brown on all sides. Transfer them to the lined baking sheet and place in the low oven to gently finish cooking through for 17–18 minutes.

To finish the salad, drain the quick-pickled red onion and scatter over the sliced tomato. Season with salt flakes.

Serve the kofta with the tzatziki, the warm 'pita' breads and the lovely fresh salad.

Nutty Cheese-burgers

with Pickled Cucumber

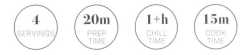

| 4 SERVINGS | 20m PREP TIME | 1+h CHILL TIME | 15m COOK TIME |

We all have our favourite burger toppings, but I wanted to create something different and fun. This super-rich topping is made from a homemade flavoured 'set' cheese to which I have added chopped nuts! Am I bonkers? Probably – but you must try it! The acidity and freshness of the Pickled Cucumber is essential to cut through the richness, finishing the burgers off nicely. Please note that the making of the Pickled Cucumber and Burger Buns are not included in the cooking times here, but they are included in the macros.

CALORIES 875 | CARBS 5.4G | FAT 74G | PROTEIN 47G

500g (1lb 2oz) minced beef, 20 per cent fat

2 tablespoons lard or ghee

4 Burger Buns (page 71)

120g (4¼oz) drained Pickled Cucumber (page 12)

lettuce (optional)

salt and freshly ground black pepper

For the nutty cheese

150g (5½oz) full-fat, mature Cheddar cheese, grated

40g (1½oz) full-fat cream cheese

1 tablespoon nutritional yeast flakes

1 teaspoon Dijon mustard

1 teaspoon apple cider vinegar

40g (1½oz) mixed roasted nuts, roughly chopped

Begin by preparing the nutty cheese. Line a 15cm (6in) square dish with clingfilm.

Place the grated cheese in a wide-bottomed microwave-safe bowl and heat in the microwave on medium for 1 minute–1 minute 30 seconds until melted. Tip into a mini food processor, then add the cream cheese, nutritional yeast flakes, mustard and vinegar. Blitz until well combined, then transfer the mixture into the prepared dish. Smooth out to an even thickness (you will be slicing this into 4 squares to top your burgers). Scatter over the chopped nuts and gently press them into the cheese. Cover and refrigerate for at least 1 hour to firm up.

To make the patties, preheat the oven to 140°C/120°C fan/275°F/ gas mark 1 and line a large baking tray with baking paper.

Season the mince generously with salt and pepper. Divide evenly into 4 portions and use clean hands to shape them into round, flat patties.

Heat the lard or ghee in a large non-stick frying pan over a medium– high heat. Add the patties and fry for 2–3 minutes on each side until caramelised and (mostly) cooked through. Transfer to the prepared baking tray and finish cooking in the oven for 3–4 minutes.

Meanwhile, remove the dish of set cheese from the fridge and slice into 4 even-sized squares. Remove the burgers from the oven and lay a square of cheese over each one. I like to keep the patties close together so you don't lose too much cheese when it melts. Return the tray to the oven for 2–3 minutes until the cheese melts.

Layer up your burgers in the Burger Buns, using lettuce if you like, along with the all-important Pickled Cucumber. Enjoy with your favourite low-carb beer (obviously!).

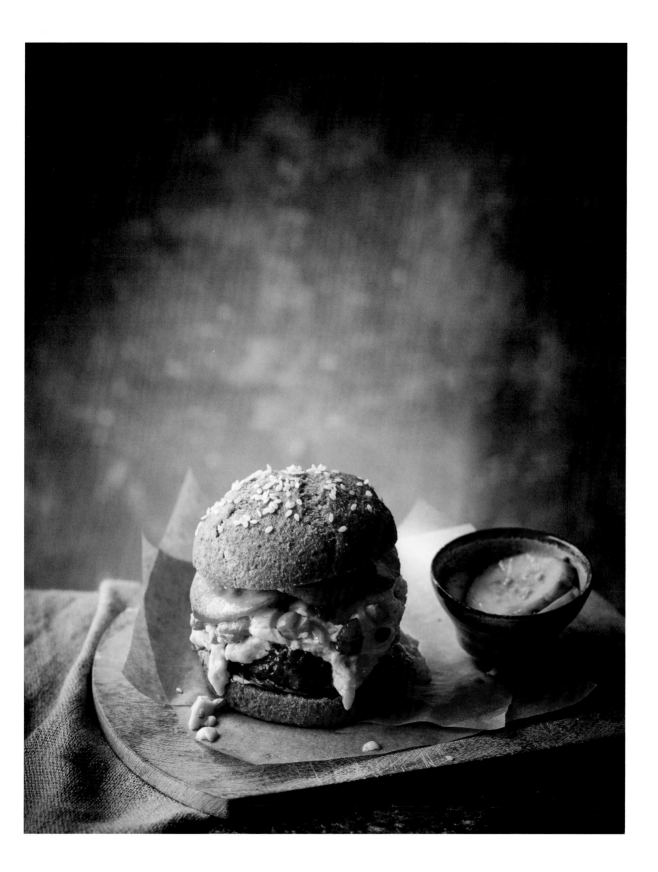

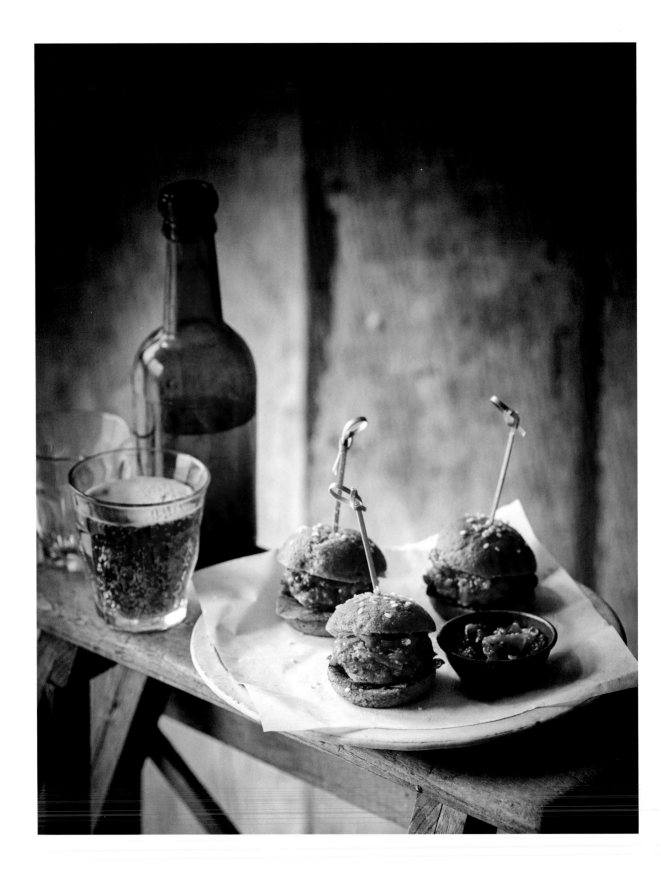

Mini Pork Sliders

with Caramelised Onion Mustard

Pork mince tends to be quite lean, so to add a more unctuous mouthfeel, I created smaller burgers with a caramelised onion and mustard topping – plus I melted slices of my Caramelised Sweet Onion Butter over each one. This recipe makes 12 miniature burgers, meaning four people can enjoy three each. The timings exclude all the premade goodies, so please bear that in mind when planning. I love the pepperiness the watercress leaves bring, but wild rocket also works.

4 SERVINGS   **25m** PREP TIME   **30m** COOK TIME

PER 3 SLIDERS: CALORIES 778 | CARBS 9.2G | FAT 67G | PROTEIN 36G

500g (1lb 2oz) minced pork (12 per cent fat)

2 teaspoons dried sage

1 teaspoon garlic powder

¼ teaspoon ground allspice

2 tablespoons lard or ghee

6 discs of Caramelised Sweet Onion Butter (page 17), halved, at room temperature

12 Mini Bread Rolls (page 108, see Tip), buttered if you like

handful of fresh watercress or wild rocket

salt flakes, salt, white pepper and freshly ground black pepper

For the caramelised onion & mustard relish

30g (1oz) unsalted butter

1 onion, thinly sliced

2 tablespoons wholegrain mustard

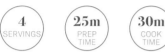

There is no need to include the thyme when you make your Mini Bread Rolls for this recipe. Instead, why not scatter over some sesame seeds before baking?

To make the caramelised onion and mustard relish, melt the butter in a frying pan over a low–medium heat. Add the onion and cook, stirring occasionally until it has completely softened and is starting to turn golden. This can take up to 25 minutes. Once you have a dark, jammy consistency, stir through the mustard, then set aside to keep warm.

Preheat the oven to 120°C/100°C fan/250°F/gas mark ½ and line a baking tray with baking paper. Combine the pork mince, sage, garlic powder and allspice in a large bowl. Season generously with salt, white pepper and freshly ground black pepper. Mix well to combine, then divide into 12 equal-sized portions (see Tip on page 63) and form into patties.

Melt the lard or ghee in a large non-stick frying pan over a high heat and fry the miniature patties for 1–2 minutes on each side until golden. Pork can very quickly dry out, so don't cook them for too long. Transfer them to the lined baking tray and leave in the warm oven until you are ready to eat.

To serve, pop half a disc of Caramelised Sweet Onion Butter on to each patty and allow to melt. Then layer up your mini bread rolls with the watercress (or rocket) leaves, followed by the patties, then some of the caramelised onion and mustard relish. Scatter over some salt flakes, if needed, and top with the mini bread roll tops. SO cute!

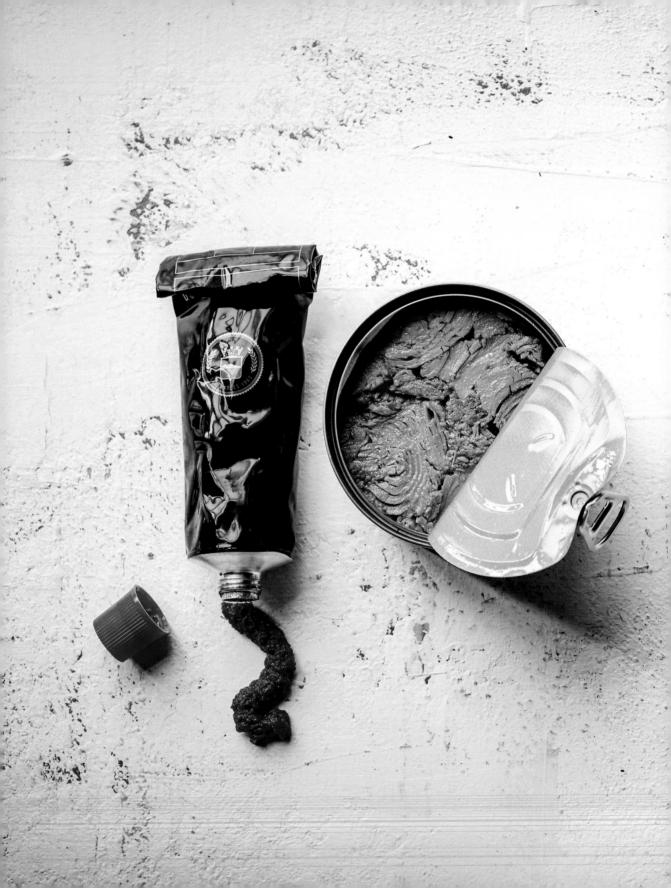

Fridge Foraging & Pantry Raiding

There are many nights when I haven't planned a dish and have to raid the fridge and pantry to see what can be used up. In all honesty, these meals are often my favourite ones.

I am thrilled with the collection of tasty recipes in this chapter. The meat and fish featured are inexpensive, and you will be surprised at the kinds of meals you can throw together with just a little imagination. If you have canned foods in your pantry (like tuna or salmon), there are some great ways to use them up other than in a sad, soggy salad.

I think I have equipped you with many wonderful ideas in this chapter, where you will learn about creative flavour combinations as well as discovering some handy cooking techniques. In fact, I'm sure that before too long, you will become so confident in the kitchen that you won't even need to refer to a recipe!

Remember, this book is not only for those on a tight budget. If you are feeling flush, replace the more affordable cuts of meat or fish with your preferred ones.

So, be inspired… and have fun!

Delicious and boasting a slight hint of spice, these celeriac chips are a great side dish option to enjoy on your low-carb journey, coming in at only 3.1g carbs per serving! They will bring back all the nostalgic memories of devouring chips – it almost feels too naughty! Why not make chip butties? If you choose to do that (using my Burger Buns, opposite), the macros for four chip butties come in at 398 calories, 7g carbs, 30g fat and 14g protein... not too shabby at all!

CALORIES 106 | CARBS 3.1G | FAT 7.9G | PROTEIN 3G

Parmesan Celeriac Chips

4 SERVINGS

10m PREP TIME

35m COOK TIME

500g (1lb 2oz) celeriac, peeled and cut intro chips approx. 1.5cm/⁵⁄₈in thick (trimmed weight)

25g (1oz) ghee or lard

½ teaspoon paprika

½ teaspoon garlic powder

15g (½oz) Parmesan or Pecorino cheese, finely grated

small handful of fresh flat-leaf parsley leaves, finely chopped

salt flakes and freshly ground black pepper

Preheat the oven to 200°C/180°C fan/400°F/gas mark 6 and line a baking tray with baking paper.

Bring a large pot of salted water to the boil and cook the celeriac chips for 3-4 minutes. You only want to partially cook them at this stage. Drain in a colander and allow to steam off completely, then spread them out on paper towels and pat dry.

Meanwhile, melt the ghee or lard in a small saucepan over a medium heat and whisk in the paprika and garlic powder. Take off the heat.

Place the cooled, dry celeriac chips in a large bowl and pour the flavoured ghee or lard over the top. Toss gently to evenly coat, then spread out on the prepared baking tray. Bake for 25–30 minutes, then scatter over three-quarters of the grated Parmesan. Return to the oven for an additional 5 minutes, cranking the heat up to maximum for the last minute.

Serve immediately, seasoned with salt flakes, freshly ground black pepper and scattered with the remaining Parmesan and a little finely chopped parsley.

*

Celeriac chips will never crisp up quite like French fries, because celeriac does not contain as much starch as potatoes, so don't worry if they don't have that crunch.

Burger Buns!

4 BUNS   **20m** PREP TIME   **25m** COOK TIME

60ml (4 tablespoons) warm water

1 teaspoon inulin powder

10g (¼oz) dried active yeast

4 large eggs, whisked

1 tablespoon olive oil

60g (2¼oz) unsalted butter, melted

50g (1¾oz) coconut flour (see Tip)

¾ teaspoon baking powder

1 teaspoon salt

½ teaspoon garlic powder

25g (1oz) psyllium husk powder

1 teaspoon sesame seeds (optional)

✳

These are trickier to roll in warm weather. If the mixture is too sticky, just use the spoon to place 4 large mounds directly on the tray, then smooth into rounds with a small silicone spatula.

✳

You can replace the coconut flour with 100g (3½oz) almond flour, but the mixture won't thicken enough to roll and shape, so you'll need to use a spoon as described on the left. This version has 3.3g carbs per bun.

Working with dried yeast is easy. If you follow the directions below, you are 45 minutes away from delicious homemade keto bread rolls. The yeast will add a delicious bready smell and flavour, but you will notice I still add a little baking powder for an extra boost. I realise you may have your own favourite low-carb rolls, but those I have seen on the market still contain vital wheat gluten, so I prefer to make my own. These are best enjoyed warm.

PER BUN: CALORIES 283 | CARBS 3.8G | FAT 22G | PROTEIN 11G

Preheat the oven to 200°C/180°C fan/400°F/gas mark 6 and line a large baking tray with baking paper.

Pour the warm water into a small bowl or ramekin. Stir in the inulin powder to dissolve. Leave to cool until tepid (hot water will kill the yeast), then scatter the yeast over the top and stir well to combine. Set aside for 15 minutes until the surface is frothy and the mixture has grown significantly in size.

In a second, medium-sized bowl, whisk together the eggs and olive oil. Once the melted butter has cooled a little, whisk this in too. In a third, large bowl, combine the coconut flour, baking powder, salt and garlic powder very well, ensuring there are no lumps.

Once the yeast mixture has visibly activated, tip it into the egg mixture and whisk well to combine, then pour this mixture into the bowl of coconut flour, whisking to create a smooth batter – it should resemble a thick custard. Add the psyllium husk powder, then immediately whisk vigorously – you have to work fast, because the psyllium will get to work very quickly thickening the mixture. Once combined, set the bowl aside for 2 minutes to stiffen and thicken further.

After 2 minutes, working quickly, use a large serving spoon to portion the mixture into 4 large, even-sized mounds and place on the prepared tray. The portions will be very soft, but can still be gently 'rolled' into a bun shape using your hands. Use a small silicone spatula to smooth their perimeters, but do not flatten the domes. Scatter over the sesame seeds (if using).

Bake on the lowest rack for 8 minutes, then reduce the oven temperature to 170°C/150°C fan/340°C/gas mark 3½ and bake for another 15–16 minutes. I always quickly rotate my tray halfway through, and I also advise laying a sheet of foil over the buns halfway through to prevent the tops darkening too much.

Soft Tortilla Wraps

(**4** WRAPS) (**30m** PREP TIME) (**15m** COOK TIME)

325g (11½oz) warm water

1 teaspoon inulin powder

10g (¼oz) dried active yeast

110g (3¾ oz) coconut flour

3 tablespoons psyllium husk powder

½ teaspoon salt

2 tablespoons olive oil

4 teaspoons ghee or lard

ground white pepper

I make these wraps often and I can assure you: practice does make perfect! These wraps are very versatile and have a delicious, bread-like aroma. I call for them in my Greek Lamb Wraps (page 36), and I have offered more of my favourite filling ideas here. In the macros, I have allowed for about 10g (¼oz) 'wasted' dough from trimming each one.

PER WRAP: CALORIES 217 | CARBS 5.2G | FAT 15G | PROTEIN 6.7G

Pour the warm water into a medium bowl and stir in the inulin powder to dissolve. Leave the water to cool until tepid, then scatter the yeast over the top and stir well. Set aside for 15 minutes until the surface is frothy and the mixture has grown significantly in size.

Combine the coconut flour, psyllium husk powder and salt in a large bowl. Season with a generous pinch of ground white pepper.

Whisk the olive oil into the yeast mixture until emulsified, then pour this wet mixture into the dry mixture, using a wooden spoon to quickly combine (the psyllium husk powder will stiffen the mixture rapidly). Smooth over and cover the surface directly with clingfilm to keep it from drying out. Set aside for 2–3 minutes.

Divide the dough into 4 equal-size portions, about 120g (4¼oz) each. Roll each one into a ball and place the first ball on a large silicone mat. Cover with a sheet of baking paper, and use a rolling pin to roll into a large circle, no bigger than 22cm (8½in) in diameter (keep the remaining dough balls covered at all times to prevent them drying out). Gently peel off the parchment, then trim around the edges to remove any jagged bits to create a beautiful disc. There shouldn't be too much in the way of off-cuts, so aim for a nice round wrap when rolling.

Heat 1 teaspoon of the ghee or lard in your largest non-stick pan (mine was 30cm/12in in diameter) over a medium–high heat, wiping the melted fat around the pan with a paper towel. Place the silicone mat upside down on one of your forearms (roll up those sleeves!) and gently peel the silicone away. Quickly place the dough disc into the pan. Cook for 1 minute 30 seconds, then use a large spatula to quickly and carefully flip and cook the underside for another 1 minute 30 seconds. Set aside and repeat with the remaining dough balls and ghee or lard. These are best enjoyed warm.

OTHER IDEAS FOR SOFT TORTILLA WRAPS

For Chicken, Avo & Tamari Mayo Wraps, mix 1 tablespoon tamari with 80g (2¾oz) mayonnaise and divide between 4 wraps. Divide 200g (7oz) cooked, sliced chicken breast, 1 sliced avocado and 1 sliced tomato between the wraps, then scatter over some fresh coriander and roll.

MAKES 4 WRAPS AT 7G CARBS EACH

For Egg & Tomato Coriander Salsa Wraps, combine 1 finely chopped tomato with ½ finely chopped red onion. Season and leave to drain in a sieve. Add a handful of chopped coriander. Scramble 8 large eggs in 2 teaspoons butter with plenty of salt and pepper. Use the eggs and salsa as fillings for the wraps.

MAKES 4 WRAPS AT 8.2G CARBS EACH

For Corned Beef & Egg Wraps, fry ½ finely chopped onion in 1 tablespoon butter until soft. Add 270g (9½oz) diced corned beef and cook until browned, then set aside. Scramble 6 large eggs in 2 teaspoons butter and season with pepper. Drizzle 4 wraps with 2 tablespoons no-added-sugar ketchup, then top with the scrambled eggs and corned beef mixture.

MAKES 4 WRAPS AT 8.9G CARBS EACH

73

Curried Tuna Salad

with Watercress & Almonds

Tuna salads tend to remind me of Life Before Keto, when I was still calorie-counting, so I wanted to give them a little flavour boost. You will notice here I use a combination of watercress and salad leaves, because the pepperiness of using only watercress can be overpowering. The macros are based on serving four people enjoying this as an easy, tasty lunch option! *Pictured on page 77.*

4 SERVINGS | **30m** PICKLE TIME | **10m** PREP TIME | **5m** COOK TIME

CALORIES 471 | CARBS 2.5G | FAT 39G | PROTEIN 27G

½ red onion, very thinly sliced

2 tablespoons apple cider vinegar

15g (½oz) flaked almonds

390g (13¾oz) canned tuna in brine (drained weight)

150g (5½oz) mayonnaise

1 tablespoon curry powder

squeeze of fresh lemon juice, to taste

90g (3¼oz) watercress

90g (3¼oz) salad leaves of your choice

2 tablespoons olive oil

small handful of fresh chives, snipped (optional)

salt and freshly ground black pepper

Place the onion in a small bowl and pour over the vinegar. Cover and leave to 'pickle' at room temperature for at least 30 minutes. Stir the mixture every now and then to ensure even pickling.

Toast the flaked almonds in a hot, dry pan over a medium heat for 1–2 minutes or until golden and toasted. Shake the pan regularly and keep your eye on them, because they can quickly burn. Set aside.

In a bowl, combine the drained tuna with the mayonnaise and curry powder. Add a squeeze of lemon juice and season with salt and pepper.

Just before serving, toss the watercress and salad leaves in the olive oil and serve with the creamy tuna mixture on top (or folded through, if you prefer). Drain the quick-pickled red onion and scatter over the top, along with the toasted almonds and snipped chives (if using).

*

Try swapping the pickled red onion for a few pieces of drained Pickled Cauliflower (page 14) for incredible bursts of acidity along with texture and crunch.

Tuna Avo Boats

with Chilli, Lime & Tamari Mayo

It beggars belief that something as simple as canned tuna could create a 'salad' as delicious as this one! It's hard to say which part is my favourite – the fatty avocado? The kick of chilli? The acidity of the lime? – but I think it's the incredible tamari-spiked mayonnaise. On a trip to Vietnam many years ago, I hounded a local family to find out why their salad dressing was so delicious: turns out it was simply a combination of tamari and mayo! *Pictured on page 76.*

4 SERVINGS **10m** PREP TIME

CALORIES 354 | CARBS 2.3G | FAT 29G | PROTEIN 18G

260g (9¼oz) canned tuna in brine (drained weight)

60g (2¼oz) mayonnaise

1 tablespoon tamari (gluten-free soy sauce) – see Tip

1 red chilli, finely chopped

finely grated zest and juice of 1 lime

4 handfuls of salad leaves

1 tablespoon olive oil

2 avocados, halved

freshly ground black pepper

In a bowl, combine the tuna, mayonnaise, tamari, chilli, lime zest and a little lime juice. Season with freshly ground black pepper. In a second bowl, toss the salad leaves in the olive oil.

Divide the salad leaves between 4 plates. Squeeze a little more lime juice over the halved avocados (this prevents them blackening), then season with freshly ground black pepper and place on top of the salad leaves before generously piling the tuna mixture on top.

If you aren't up for the hassle of eating this salad as indicated here, simply dice the avocados and add them to the delicious tuna mixture before serving over the dressed salad leaves.

If you have soy allergies or prefer to omit soy on your keto journey, use coconut aminos instead, which offers a similar flavour. I love tamari on occasion, so I guess that makes me a little 'dirty' keto!

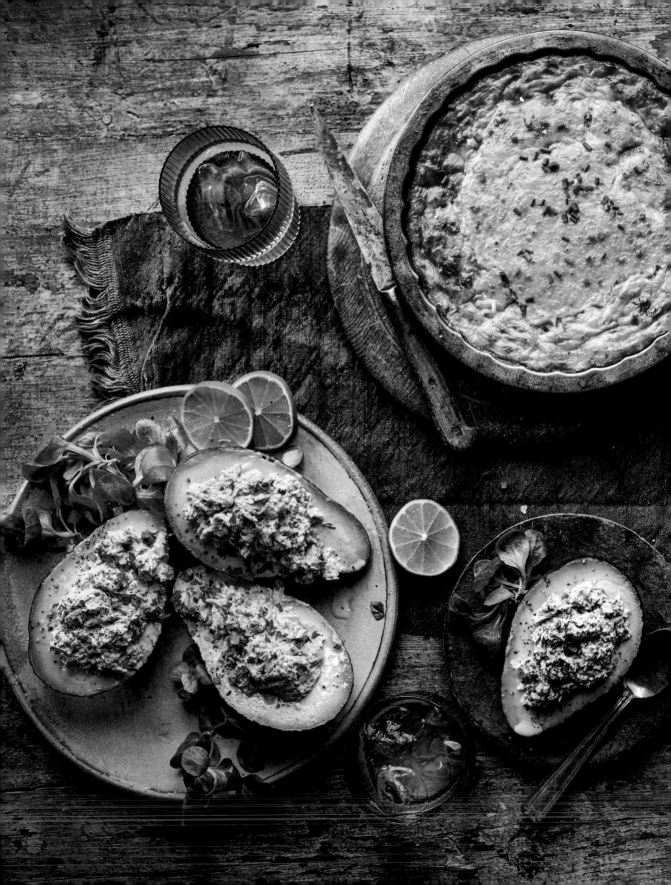

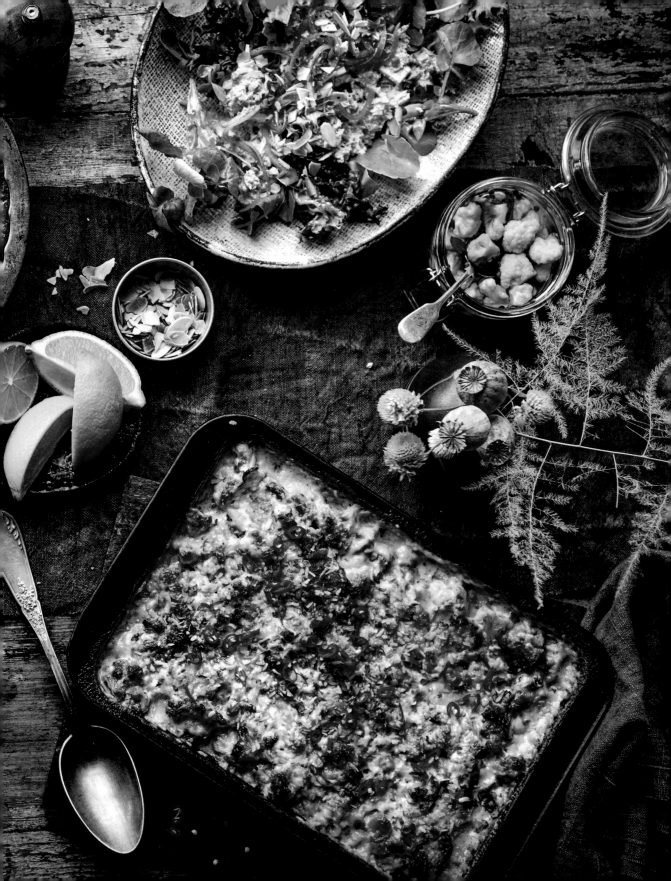

Cheesy Tuna & Tomato Quiche

Another superb thing to do with canned tuna! This crustless quiche can be sliced into eight, and I advise you to serve two slices per person (serving four), because it is just so flavour-packed and moreish! I used Gruyère cheese here, which can be a little pricier, but leftover Gruyère can still be put to good use: try dicing it up and enjoying it with some Pickled Baby Onions (page 14) for a late-afternoon snack. Enjoy this quiche with a lovely green salad on the side. *Pictured on page 76.*

4 SERVINGS | **20m** PREP TIME | **50m** COOK TIME

1 tablespoon unsalted butter

2 tomatoes, finely chopped

1 garlic clove, finely chopped

1 tablespoon double-concentrated tomato purée

130g (4¾oz) canned tuna in brine (drained weight)

100g (3½oz) full-fat cream cheese

50g (1¾oz) Gruyère cheese, finely grated

3 large eggs

180ml (6fl oz) double cream

salt flakes, salt and ground white pepper

CALORIES 461 | CARBS 4.5G | FAT 40G | PROTEIN 19G

Preheat the oven to 200°C/180°C fan/400°F/gas mark 6. Grease an 18cm (7in) loose-bottomed tart tin. Line the base (and a little way up the sides) with baking paper, then place the tin on a baking tray. (Letting the baking paper come up the sides just a little helps to avoid the mixture leaking out the bottom, which can often happen with loose-bottomed tart tins.)

Melt the butter in a small non-stick saucepan over a medium heat. Add the tomatoes, garlic and tomato purée and cook for 8–9 minutes until the tomatoes break down and the excess moisture cooks out. By this time, the garlic will have sufficiently softened, too.

Tip the mixture into a medium bowl and add the tuna and cream cheese (ensure the tuna is drained well to prevent a watery quiche). Set aside for 5 minutes to cool a little, then stir through the grated cheese. Season with salt and pepper.

In a separate, larger bowl, whisk together the eggs and double cream. Add the tuna and tomato mixture and combine well. Pour the mixture into the prepared tin, then transfer to the oven (still on the baking tray) and bake for 25 minutes. (I like to rotate the tray halfway through to ensure even baking.)

After 25 minutes, turn the oven off and leave the door slightly ajar to allow the quiche to gently finish cooking in the residual heat for another 15 minutes.

Remove from the oven and allow to cool slightly, then use the back of a teaspoon to nudge the edges of the tin if any mixture is stuck. Slice and serve. Simple and truly delicious!

Coconut Cauliflower Bake

with Canned Salmon

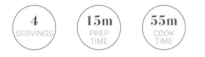

4 SERVINGS | **15m** PREP TIME | **55m** COOK TIME

500g (1lb 2oz) cauliflower , chopped into small, even-sized pieces

50g (1¾oz) coconut oil, melted

400g (14oz) can full-fat coconut milk

3 garlic cloves, roughly chopped

25g (1oz) fresh root ginger, peeled and roughly chopped

1 lemongrass stalk, roughly chopped (hard outer layer discarded)

1 lime, zested then cut into 4 wedges

100ml (3½fl oz) double cream

1 teaspoon desiccated coconut

250g (9oz) canned salmon, drained (drained weight)

salt and ground white pepper

To finish

2 tablespoons desiccated coconut

1 red chilli, sliced

small handful of fresh coriander leaves, finely chopped

salt flakes (if needed)

This is a beautiful little invention, and one of many recipes in this book that I absolutely love and now make often. The flavours are massive and a great way to use up any garlic, lemongrass and ginger you may have kicking about. If you are feeling a little 'flush', then by all means use fresh salmon – simply chop it and follow the recipe as below, although you may need to add another 4–5 minutes to the baking time. This is delicious served as is, but I love it over courgetti, or even with Burger Buns (page 71) to mop up the dreamy sauce! *Pictured on page 77.*

CALORIES 573 | CARBS 9.2G | FAT 51G | PROTEIN 21G

Preheat the oven to 200°C/180°C fan/400°F/gas mark 6 and grease a large baking tray (or line with baking paper) .

Place the cauliflower in a large bowl and pour over the melted coconut oil. Lightly salt the mixture and toss well to evenly coat. Spread out on the prepared baking tray and bake for 24–25 minutes until golden. Remove from the oven and set aside for now. Do not turn the oven off.

Meanwhile, add the coconut milk to a mini food processor or food chopper, along with the garlic, ginger and lemongrass. Blitz very well, stopping every now and then to scrape down the sides. Tip the mixture into a large non-stick pan or wok over a high heat. Add the lime zest, cream and 1 teaspoon desiccated coconut. Bring the mixture to the boil, then reduce the heat to low and simmer for 9–10 minutes until the mixture reduces to a thicker consistency, stirring occasionally.

Remove the pan from the heat and stir in the salmon and the roasted cauliflower florets. Season generously with salt and ground white pepper and mix well to combine before tipping the whole lot into a deep 16 x 25cm (6¼ x 10in) roasting dish. Bake for 25–30 minutes until the creamy mix has baked down and thickened.

Meanwhile, toast the desiccated coconut in a dry pan over a medium heat for 2–3 minutes until golden. Stir continuously and keep your eye on the pan, because desiccated coconut can quickly burn. Set aside to use as garnish.

Serve the bake garnished with the toasted coconut, red chilli and coriander. Serve with the lime wedges for squeezing, to enhance the acidity (if you feel it needs it). Add some salt flakes, too, if you like. Delicious!

Fish
with Browned Butter & Capers

This simple dinner requires very little effort and offers a delicious and interesting way to spruce up your white fish. The capers add great little bursts of salty flavour, while the browned butter and lemon make the end result irresistible. Delicious with your favourite vegetables on the side – we love it with a simple bowl of chopped tomatoes, dressed with a little olive oil and crushed garlic stirred in.

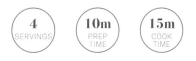

4 SERVINGS   **10m** PREP TIME   **15m** COOK TIME

CALORIES 280 | CARBS <0.5G | FAT 21G | PROTEIN 22G

4 skinless white fish fillets (approx. 125g/4½oz each)

1 tablespoon olive oil

70g (2½oz) unsalted butter

3 garlic cloves, smashed with the back of a knife

10g (¼oz) small capers, drained (about 1 heaped tablespoon)

salt and ground white pepper

freshly squeezed lemon juice, to finish

small handful of freshly snipped chives, to garnish

Preheat the oven to 200°C/180°C fan/400°F/gas mark 6 and line a baking tray with baking paper.

Remove the fish fillets from the packaging and pat dry with a paper towel. Place them on the prepared baking tray. Season with a little salt and ground white pepper, then drizzle or brush over the olive oil. Bake for 10–11 minutes until the fish is cooked and flakes easily.

Meanwhile, heat 60g (2¼oz) of the butter in a saucepan over a medium heat and leave to melt. Once it starts to foam, add the smashed garlic cloves. The milk solids in the butter will start to brown, adding further to the beautiful aroma. This will take about 5–7 minutes.

Remove the pan from the heat and pour the contents through a sieve lined with muslin or cheesecloth and into a small, clean saucepan. Discard the browned milk solids and garlic caught in the muslin.

Place the clean pan of browned, garlic-infused butter over a low heat. Add the remaining butter, along with the capers, and leave on the heat until all the butter has melted.

This should have melted and warmed through at around the same time the fish in the oven has cooked through.

Serve the cooked fish with the warm browned butter poured over the top. The capers will add enough saltiness, so just a crack of black pepper and a good squeeze of fresh lemon juice will finish the dish perfectly. Scatter the chives over the top and enjoy with your favourite vegetables or salad.

*

You could skip making the browned butter here and simply use 60g (2¼oz) of Garlic-infused Browned Butter (page 18) if you have some already made.

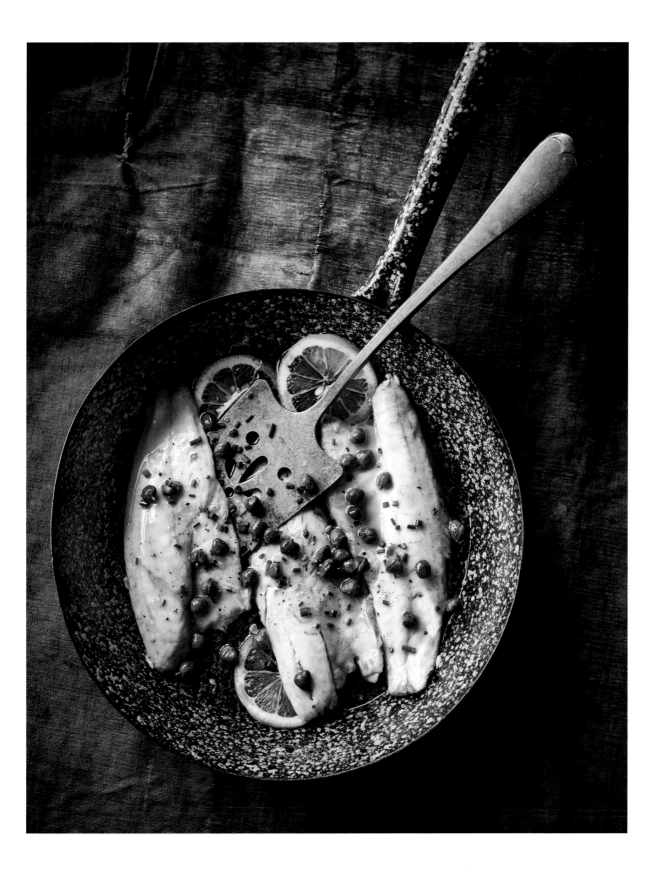

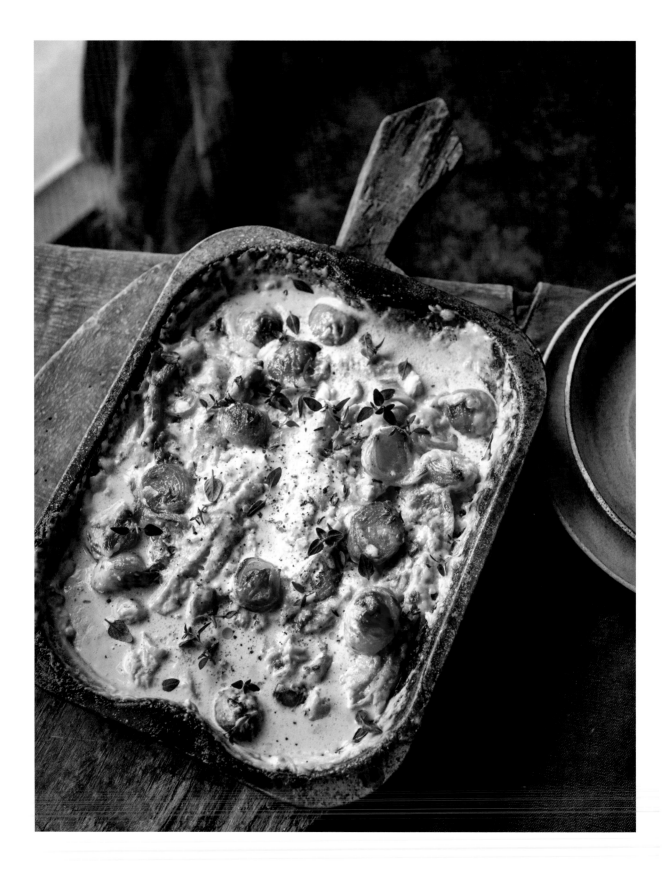

Creamy Baked Fish

with Baby Onions & Thyme

This is a simply scrumptious fish dinner where a garlic and thyme-infused cream bakes down to create a glorious flavour. The baby onions add just a hint of sweetness, and if you find yourself with half a bag of baby onions left over after making this dish, why not use them to make the Pickled Onions on page 14? That's what I do!

4 SERVINGS | **10m** PREP TIME | **40m** COOK TIME

CALORIES 427 | CARBS 4.4G | FAT 35G | PROTEIN 22G

150g (5½oz) baby onions or round shallots, halved through the root (see Tip for easy peeling)

1 teaspoon olive oil

1 teaspoon unsalted butter

3 garlic cloves, finely chopped

3–4 fresh thyme sprigs, leaves picked, plus extra to garnish

250ml (9fl oz) double cream

4 white skinless fish fillets (approx. 120g/4¼oz each)

salt flakes, salt, ground white pepper and freshly ground black pepper

*

Peeling baby onions or shallots can be frustrating. I place them in a bowl and pour over boiling hot water, then leave them to sit for 15–20 minutes. This makes them much easier to peel.

Preheat the oven to 200°C/180°C fan/400°F/gas mark 6 and grease a small roasting dish (it should be the right size to allow all 4 fish fillets to sit snugly together when we add them later).

Place the onions in the prepared roasting dish and drizzle over the olive oil, then toss to coat. Roast for 15 minutes.

Meanwhile, melt the butter in a saucepan over a medium heat. Add the garlic and cook for 1–2 minutes until softened. Add the thyme leaves and cream and bring to a simmer for 3–4 minutes, allowing the cream to reduce a little. This will give you maximum infusion of flavour from the garlic and thyme. Season with salt and ground white pepper.

Once the onions are done, remove them from the oven and tip them into the pan of simmering cream. You will use the roasting dish again, so set it aside for now.

Remove the fish fillets from their packaging and lightly season all sides with salt and ground white pepper. Lay them in the roasting dish, then pour the creamy onion mixture over the top, nestling the onions in between the fish. Bake for 23–24 minutes.

Season with salt flakes and freshly ground black pepper, and serve with more picked thyme leaves scattered over the top. I like to flake the fish right there in the pan after baking and serve over Creamy Cauliflower Rice (page 29) or courgetti.

Fish & Mixed Pepper Turmeric Stew

4 SERVINGS | **15m** PREP TIME | **30m** COOK TIME

2 tablespoons unsalted butter

1 red pepper, diced small

1 yellow pepper, diced small

2 garlic cloves, finely chopped

juice of 1 lemon

1 teaspoon ground turmeric

300ml (10fl oz) fish stock

600g (1lb 5oz) skinless, deboned white fish, cut into bite-sized chunks

60g (2¼oz) soured cream

handful of fresh coriander leaves, finely chopped

salt and ground white pepper

*

Blitzing half the cooked vegetables adds 'body' to thicken the mixture, while keeping some whole adds colour and texture to the dish.

This fish dish is a hearty, beautiful meal in the chillier months. Like most things, it can be frozen, but I advise you to add the soured cream and fresh coriander just before serving. You will notice that it is pretty low in fat, but we love it over the delicious Creamy Cauliflower Rice (page 29), which is enriched with butter, cream cheese and double cream – perfect!

CALORIES 224 | CARBS 4.2G | FAT 10G | PROTEIN 29G

Melt the butter in a large non-stick saucepan over a medium heat. Fry the peppers for 4–5 minutes until they start to soften. Add the garlic and continue to cook for another 1–2 minutes until the garlic softens and the peppers begin to caramelise. Stir regularly to avoid the garlic burning. Deglaze the pan with the lemon juice (catch the pips!) and cook until the lemon juice completely evaporates. Use a slotted spoon to remove half of the cooked mixture and set it aside in a small bowl for now.

Add the turmeric to the mixture still in the pan and cook for 1 minute before pouring in the fish stock. Increase the heat and bring to the boil, then remove the pan from the heat and use a hand blender, right there in the pan, to blitz the mixture until smooth (tipping the pan to one side helps). Return the pan to a medium heat and allow the mixture to reduce to create a thicker sauce (see Tip). This can take up to 5 minutes.

Add the batch of diced peppers you set aside earlier, along with the fish chunks. Reduce the heat to medium–low and cook for 14–15 minutes, stirring occasionally, to allow the fish to gently poach in the mixture. Season with salt and ground white pepper and stir through the soured cream just before serving, then scatter over the coriander.

Serve over your choice of 'base'. We love it with the Creamy Cauliflower Rice (page 29) as pictured (not included in the macros), with some Curry Butter (page 17) stirred through.

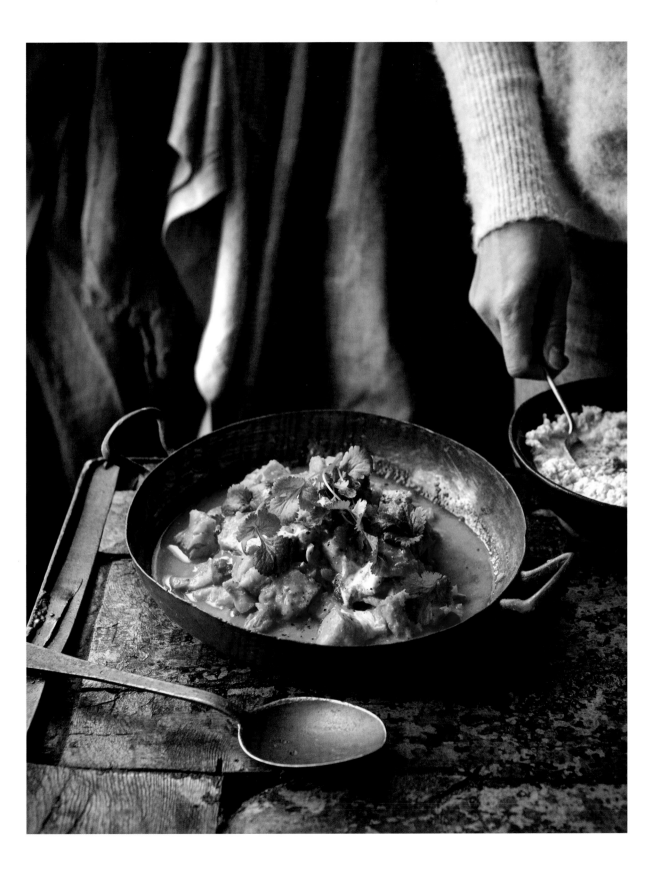

Chicken Livers

in Brandy Tomato Cream

This is a small nod to eating nose-to-tail – or, in the case of chicken, maybe that should be beak-to-tail (although I should clarify, there are no beaks here!). I adore chicken livers: not only are they incredibly affordable, but liver is a very nutrient-dense food. I love them spicy (like the recipe in my first book, *Keto Kitchen*), but this creamy tomato mixture is equally fantastic. The brandy flavour is subtle, but still beautifully evident.

| 4 SERVINGS | 20m PREP TIME | 45m COOK TIME |

CALORIES 557 | CARBS 8.2G | FAT 36G | PROTEIN 48G

400g (14oz) can chopped tomatoes

750g (1lb 10oz) chicken livers (trimmed weight)

3 tablespoons unsalted butter

1 onion, thinly sliced

3 garlic cloves, finely chopped

60ml (4 tablespoons) brandy

1 tablespoon double-concentrated tomato purée

130ml (4½fl oz) double cream

50g (1¾oz) soured cream

3–4 fresh thyme sprigs, leaves picked

salt flakes, salt and freshly ground black pepper

*

Like all meat, the surface of the livers should be as dry as possible before cooking to ensure the best caramelisation.

Blitz the tomatoes in a mini food processor or food chopper until smooth. Set aside.

Drain the chicken livers in a colander before using (see Tip). Remove and discard the sinewy bits, then cut the livers into small, even-sized pieces and pat dry. Melt 1 tablespoon of the butter in a large, non-stick frying pan over a high heat. Fry half the livers for 2–3 minutes until golden and caramelised on all sides. Be careful – some of the pieces might pop out of the pan! Transfer to a bowl and season with salt. Repeat with another 1 tablespoon of butter and the remaining livers. Don't worry if they're not cooked through yet – they will be later. (Cooking the livers in batches is important to achieve the high-heat browning needed here, which isn't possible in an overcrowded pan.)

Return the empty pan to the hob and reduce the heat to medium. Melt the remaining 1 tablespoon of butter in the pan, then add the onion and cook for 10–11 minutes until softened. Add the garlic and cook for 1–2 minutes, stirring continuously as the onion starts to caramelise. Pour in the brandy, which will deglaze the pan. Use your spatula to scrape the pan to loosen any bits that are stuck. Once all the brandy has evaporated, add the blitzed tomato mixture and tomato purée and stir through. Leave to simmer over a medium heat for 12–15 minutes until the mixture has reduced to a thick sauce.

Return the livers to the pan (along with any resting juices from the bowl) and simmer for 4–5 minutes. I like my livers pink, but if you prefer them cooked more, leave them on the heat for longer. Add the cream and soured cream and cook for another 4–5 minutes to gently warm through and thicken. Season generously with salt flakes and black pepper, and serve garnished with freshly picked thyme leaves.

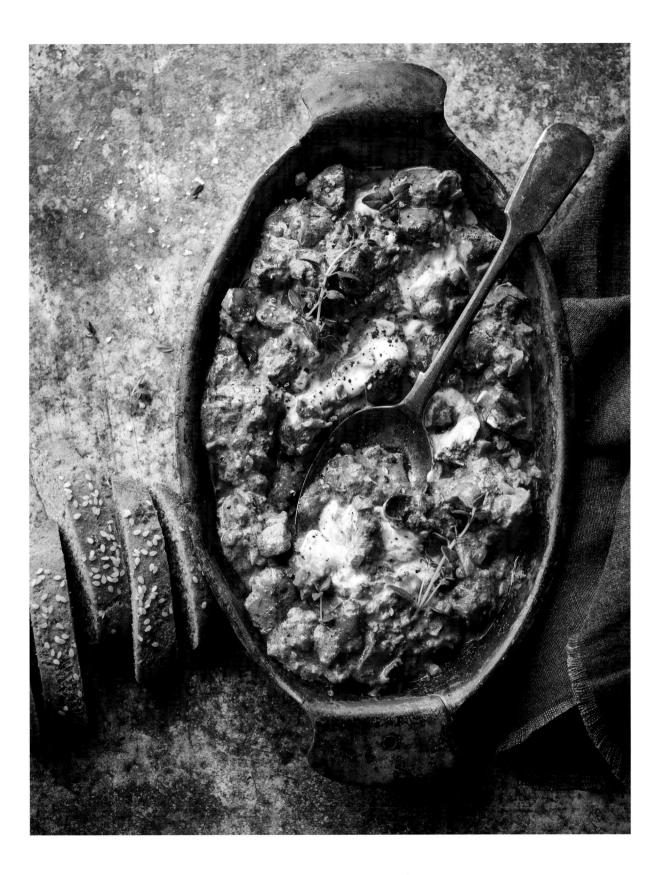

Spicy Wings
Two Ways

with Two Dipping Options

4 SERVINGS

20m PREP TIME

30m COOK TIME

Chicken wings are inexpensive and always a crowd-pleaser. I have offered two different ways to spice them up, and there are two fantastic dipping sauce options to choose from. The wings can be shared between four people as part of a main meal, or perhaps as a lighter meal or appetiser. Enjoy these with your favourite vegetables or salad on the side. The macros given for the wings exclude any dips, and the macros given for the dips exclude any wings.

OPTION 1: CALORIES 679 | CARBS 3.4G | FAT 47G | PROTEIN 59G

OPTION 2: CALORIES 635 | CARBS 2.1G | FAT 43G | PROTEIN 58G

Option 1 – Ketchup & Tamari

1kg (2lb 4oz) chicken wings

1 teaspoon garlic powder

1 teaspoon cayenne pepper

90g (3¼oz) no-added-sugar ketchup

2 tablespoons tamari (gluten-free soy sauce)

1 tablespoon olive oil

2 teaspoons Dijon mustard

handful of any fresh herbs, finely chopped to garnish (optional)

salt flakes, salt, white pepper and freshly ground black pepper

Option 2 – Spicy Garlic & Paprika

1kg (2lb 4oz) chicken wings

1 teaspoon onion powder

1 teaspoon garlic powder

1 teaspoon cayenne pepper

1 teaspoon paprika

handful of any fresh herbs, finely chopped, to garnish (optional)

Preheat the oven to 200°C/180°C fan/400°F/gas mark 6.

For option 1, place the wings in a large bowl and scatter over the garlic powder, cayenne pepper and a generous seasoning of salt and pepper. In a separate small bowl, whisk together the ketchup, tamari, olive oil and mustard. Massage this sauce into the wings until evenly coated. Spread out on a large baking tray lined with baking paper and roast for about 25–30 minutes until cooked through. Season with salt flakes and freshly ground black pepper, and scatter over the chopped herbs.

For option 2, place the wings in a large bowl and scatter over the onion powder, garlic powder, cayenne pepper and paprika. Season with salt and pepper and massage the spices into the chicken. Cook as above.

Enjoy as they are or serve with your chosen dipping sauce (both dipping sauces work with either option, so the choice is yours!).

Blue Cheese Dipping Sauce

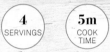

4 SERVINGS   **5m** COOK TIME

<0.5G CARBS PER SERVING

Crumble 90g (3¼oz) blue cheese into a small saucepan along with 50ml (2fl oz) double cream. Heat gently over a medium heat until the cheese completely melts and the cream warms through and reduces slightly. (This is magnificent over steak, too!)

Ranch Dressing Dip

4 SERVINGS   **5m** PREP TIME

1.5G CARBS PER SERVING

Combine 60g (2¼oz) mayonnaise, 60g (2¼oz) soured cream, 2 tablespoons double cream and 1 teaspoon apple cider vinegar in a bowl. Add ½ teaspoon each of garlic powder and onion powder, along with a handful of finely chopped flat-leaf parsley. Season with salt and pepper and mix well to combine.

Sesame Chicken

with Red Cabbage & Avo Slaw

I love crispy chicken thighs, and thoroughly enjoy them served with this scrumptious slaw, which boasts so many different flavours and textures. It also makes a great side salad – try it at your next *braai* (barbecue)! I am aware that macadamia nuts can be pricey, but I chop them smaller, meaning a little goes a long way here. I stuck to moderate protein (as keto suggests), but you may want to add more chicken pieces if you prefer.

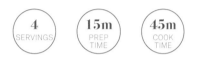

4 SERVINGS | **15m** PREP TIME | **45m** COOK TIME

CALORIES 558 | CARBS 3.9G | FAT 46G | PROTEIN 29G

4 large chicken thighs, skin-on (approx. 170g/6oz each)

½ tablespoon sesame oil, plus additional ½ tablespoon to finish

1 tablespoon sesame seeds

salt flakes, salt and freshly ground black pepper

For the caramelised nuts

30g (1oz) macadamia nuts

1 teaspoon unsalted butter

1 tablespoon sugar-free syrup

For the slaw

2 avocados, peeled and chopped

juice of 2 limes

200g (7oz) red cabbage, finely sliced

handful of fresh coriander leaves, finely chopped

handful of fresh mint leaves, finely chopped

handful of fresh flat-leaf parsley leaves, finely chopped

2 tablespoons sesame oil

*

Clean your pastry brush well after brushing the underside of the raw chicken.

Start with the caramelised nuts. Preheat the oven to 200°C/180°C fan/400°F/gas mark 6. Spread the macadamia nuts out on a small baking tray and roast for 6–7 minutes until golden. Set aside, but do not turn the oven off.

Melt the butter in a small non-stick saucepan over a high heat and tip in the roasted nuts. Add the sugar-free syrup and cook, stirring continuously to coat the nuts, for 2–3 minutes. Tip the coated nuts out on to a silicone mat or sheet of baking paper and spread out. Leave to cool completely. Once cool, roughly chop and set aside.

Use a pastry brush to lightly brush the underside of the chicken pieces with ½ tablespoon of sesame oil, then season all sides with salt. (Don't be tempted to brush the skins prior to roasting, because they may not crisp up as much.) Place the chicken pieces, skin-side up, on a roasting tray and scatter over the sesame seeds. Roast in the oven for 30–35 minutes until the chicken is safely cooked through and the skins are gloriously crispy. Just before serving, use a clean pastry brush (see Tip) to lightly brush the crispy skins with another ½ tablespoon of sesame oil.

While the chicken is cooking, make the slaw. Place the chopped avocados in a bowl and generously squeeze over the lime juice. Season with salt and freshly ground black pepper. In a separate bowl, toss together the cabbage, finely chopped herbs and sesame oil.

Just before serving, add the avocado to the cabbage and scatter over the caramelised macadamia nuts. Serve the chicken with the slaw on the side, seasoning the chicken with salt flakes.

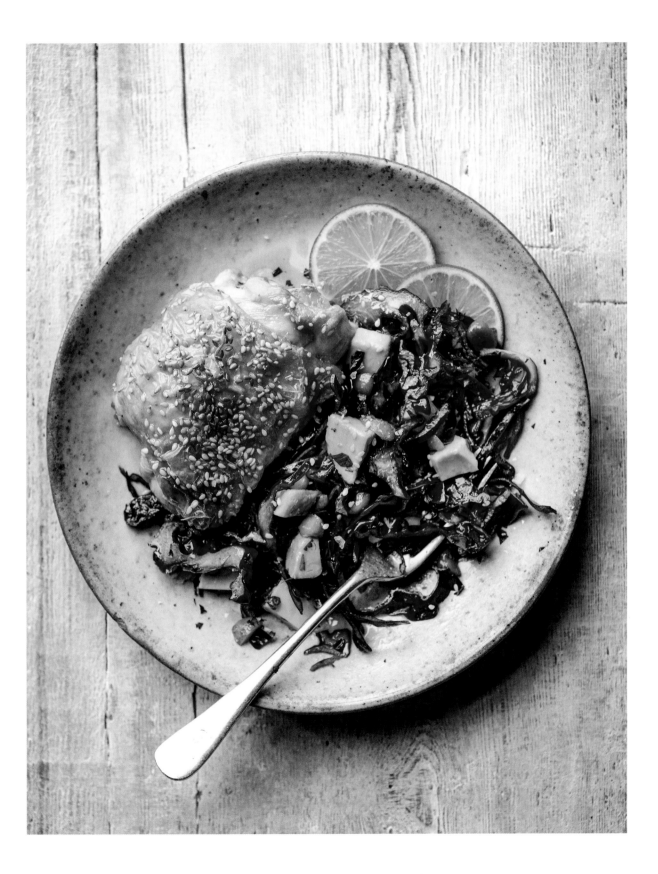

Stuffed Chicken

with Buttery Broccoli

There is always a head of broccoli kicking about in our fridge and I just love experimenting with different ways to use it. I think I love it most simply boiled until tender, then smothered in melted butter – or, in this case, the rendered fat and juices of ham-and-cheese-stuffed chicken thighs (after all, why waste fat?). These chicken thighs are like an uncomplicated cordon bleu, and taste utterly delicious. The carbs here mostly come from the broccoli, so there is no judgement from me if you want to double up on the stuffed chicken!

4 SERVINGS   **20m** PREP TIME   **35m** COOK TIME

CALORIES 387 | CARBS 3.7G | FAT 24G | PROTEIN 37G

4 large chicken thighs, skin on (approx. 170g/6oz each)

4 teaspoons Dijon mustard (see Tip)

4 generous pinches of garlic powder

50g (1¾oz) full-fat mature Cheddar cheese, finely grated

4 slices deli ham (60g/2¼oz total weight)

400g (14oz) broccoli, chopped into even-sized pieces

20g (¾oz) unsalted butter, melted

salt flakes, salt, ground white pepper and freshly ground black pepper

Preheat the oven to 200°C/180°C fan/400°F/gas mark 6.

Lift the skins from your chicken pieces as much as possible without removing them completely. This is easily done by simply lifting the skin at the edge and using a blunt butter knife to separate the 'membrane' between skin and flesh. With the skin flapped open, spread a teaspoon of mustard on to the flesh of each thigh (see Tip), followed by a scattering of ground white pepper and a generous pinch of garlic powder. Next, add a layer of grated cheese, followed by the ham, tucking them in neatly. Fold the skin back over to ensure you have a neat little parcel, free of any escaping cheese! Crack a generous amount of black pepper over the stuffed chicken thighs and place on a roasting tray (skin-side up). Roast for 30–35 minutes until the chicken is safely cooked through and the skins are crispy.

Meanwhile, bring a large pan of salted water to the boil. Add the broccoli and cook for 4–5 minutes until tender. Drain well in a colander and place in a serving dish. Pour over the melted butter, then cover with foil and set aside to keep warm.

Once the chicken is ready, gently remove from the oven and transfer the thighs to 4 plates. In the roasting tray, there will be plenty of fat, juices and some escaped melted cheese – pour this over the broccoli, then divide between the plates.

Season with salt flakes and freshly ground black pepper (if you feel the dish needs it), and serve.

*

Portion out the 4 teaspoons of mustard into a small bowl before spreading on the raw chicken to prevent dangerous 'double-dipping' between raw chicken and your jar of Dijon.

*

Don't stop at Cheddar and deli ham! Try any of your favourite cheese and deli meat combinations. Gruyère and salami, anyone?

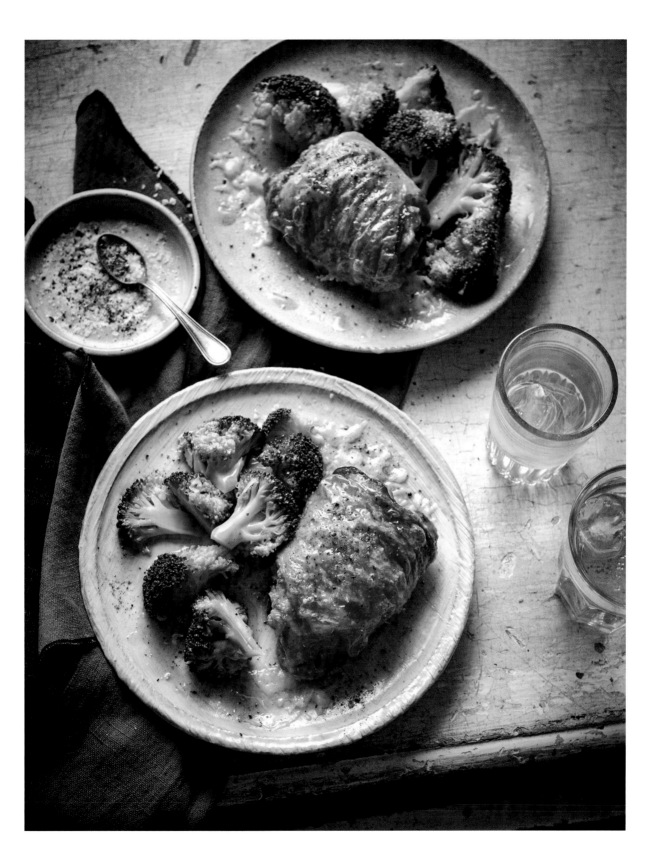

Ginger Chicken

with Coconut Spinach & Tomatoes

When I was at culinary school, a classmate shared with me how delicious chicken was when cooked with tomatoes and ginger. Years later – and still inspired by this combination – I played around with many ways to include all three elements. What resulted was this great dish, where I serve ginger-seasoned chicken pieces with a creamy coconut spinach and add tomatoes for sweet bites. This is delicious over Creamy Cauliflower Rice (page 29) or even cauliflower mash to mop up the dreamy, creamy spinach.

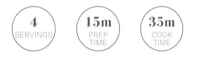

4 SERVINGS   **15m** PREP TIME   **35m** COOK TIME

CALORIES 585 | CARBS 6.9G | FAT 44G | PROTEIN 40G

8 chicken pieces (thighs and drumsticks), approx. 1.2kg (2lb 10oz) total weight

2 teaspoons ground ginger

45g (1¾oz) fresh root ginger, peeled and roughly chopped

1 lemongrass stalk, roughly chopped (hard outer layer discarded)

3 garlic cloves, roughly chopped

400g (14oz) can full-fat coconut milk

350g (12oz) baby spinach leaves

2 tomatoes, each cut into 8 wedges

salt flakes, salt and freshly ground black pepper

handful of fresh coriander or flat-leaf parsley leaves, finely chopped

Preheat the oven to 200°C/180°C fan/400°F/gas mark 6.

Season the chicken pieces on all sides with the ground ginger and a little salt. Place on a large baking tray (skin-side up) and bake for 30–35 minutes until the chicken sufficiently cooks through.

Meanwhile, place the fresh ginger, lemongrass, garlic and coconut milk in a mini food processor or food chopper. Blitz very well, scraping down the sides once or twice to ensure you have a relatively smooth mixture.

Pour this mixture into a large non-stick pan or wok over a medium heat and bring to a simmer. Once simmering, tip in all the spinach until it wilts into the warm coconut milk (you may need to add it in two batches). Once all the spinach has wilted, continue to cook for 15–18 minutes or until the coconut milk has reduced by more than half and you are left with a thick creamed spinach. Add the tomato wedges and reduce the heat to low, gently cooking for another 9–10 minutes. The tomatoes will release some moisture of their own, but we don't want to cook them too much, because they bring such a beautiful, fresh flavour to this dish.

When everything is ready, serve the delicious chicken pieces with the lovely creamed spinach mixture and garnish with chopped coriander (or parsley, if you prefer). Season with salt flakes and freshly ground black pepper if you feel it needs it.

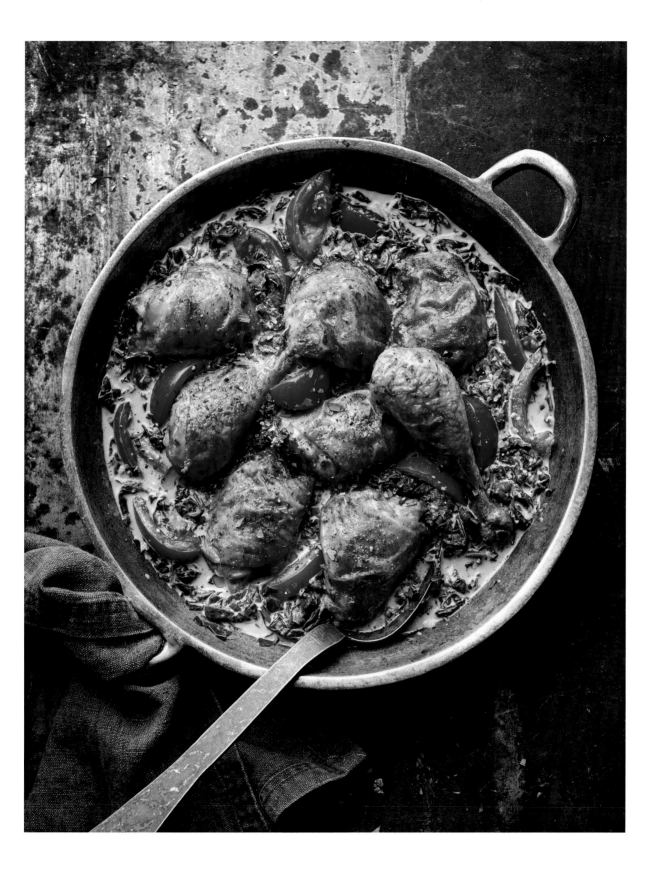

Cumin & Paprika Chicken

with Cauliflower 'Couscous'

Baking cauliflower 'couscous' in the same dish as the chicken here means it absorbs all those delicious flavours! You will love the spice mix in this recipe – and please don't skip the chopped herb garnish, which adds additional top notes and a fresh flavour. If you don't like coriander, parsley will also be lovely. *Pictured on page 98.*

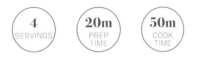

4 SERVINGS | **20m** PREP TIME | **50m** COOK TIME

CALORIES 440 | CARBS 7.3G | FAT 27G | PROTEIN 41G

8 chicken pieces (thighs and drumsticks), approx. 1.2kg (2lb 10oz) total weight

2 teaspoons ground cumin

2 teaspoons paprika

2 teaspoons garlic powder

1 red onion, cut into 8 wedges (see Tip)

1 teaspoon olive oil

handful of fresh coriander or flat-leaf parsley leaves, finely chopped

salt flakes, salt and freshly ground black pepper

For the cauliflower 'couscous'

500g (1lb 2oz) cauliflower florets

1 teaspoon ground cumin

1 teaspoon paprika

1 teaspoon garlic powder

*

Keep the root end of the onion intact when cutting into wedges: this will ensure each wedge holds together when cooking.

Preheat the oven to 200°C/180°C fan/400°F/gas mark 6.

Place the chicken pieces in a large bowl and add the cumin, paprika, garlic powder and some salt. Get stuck in with clean hands to massage the spice mix into the chicken pieces. Lay them out in a large, deep roasting dish (skin-side up). Brush the red onion wedges with the olive oil and add to the same dish. Roast in the oven for 25 minutes.

Meanwhile, blitz the cauliflower in a food processor until it resembles coarse breadcrumbs. Set aside.

Remove the dish from the oven and use tongs to remove the chicken and roasted onions, setting them aside on a large plate for now (keep the chicken skin-side up). Pour the juices and rendered fat into a large non-stick pan or wok. Keep the oven on, and keep the roasting dish at hand, as you will still use it again soon.

Add the blitzed cauliflower to the pan of rendered fat and juices, along with the cumin, paprika and garlic powder. Season with a little salt. Cook over a high heat for about 2 minutes until the cauliflower starts to soften. Stir continuously to ensure it is evenly coated in the juice and spices.

Tip the cauliflower mixture into the original roasting dish, then return the chicken pieces and partially roasted red onion wedges to the dish too, nestling them into the cauliflower 'couscous'. Return to the oven for 15–20 minutes until the chicken has safely cooked through.

Serve with freshly chopped coriander or parsley generously scattered over the top, and seasoned with some salt flakes and freshly ground black pepper if you feel it needs it.

Paprika Chicken

with Zingy Creamed Spinach

This is another great way to enjoy crispy chicken thighs. The smoked paprika flavour complements the accompanying zingy creamed spinach just beautifully. Speaking of which, this is like creamed spinach on steroids! I added everything I could imagine to enhance it, and I bet you will never consider regular creamed spinach again. So rich, so delicious, so very low in carbs... This dish is delicious when enjoyed with ripe sliced tomatoes on the side (not included in the macros) which offer sweetness and acidity to cut through the rich spinach. *Pictured on page 99.*

4 SERVINGS | **15m** PREP TIME | **55m** COOK TIME

CALORIES 534 | CARBS 2.7G | FAT 39G | PROTEIN 43G

4 large chicken thighs, skin on (approx. 170g/6oz each)

½ teaspoon smoked paprika

freshly ground black pepper

For the spinach

3 garlic cloves, finely chopped

½ teaspoon smoked paprika

juice of 1 lemon

400g (14oz) baby spinach leaves

100ml (3½fl oz) double cream

50g (1¾oz) soured cream

40g (1½oz) Parmesan or Pecorino cheese, finely grated

5–6 fresh thyme sprigs, leaves picked, plus extra to serve (optional)

salt flakes, salt and ground white pepper

Preheat the oven to 200°C/180°C fan/400°F/gas mark 6.

Place the chicken thighs in a bowl. Scatter over the smoked paprika and crack over a generous amount of freshly ground black pepper. Get stuck in with clean hands, massaging the spices into the chicken pieces so they are evenly coated. Place the chicken on a roasting tray, skin-side up, and roast for 30–35 minutes until the skins are crispy and the chicken has safely cooked through. Remove from the roasting tray and set aside to keep warm.

There should be juices and rendered fat in the roasting tray. To make the creamed spinach, pour these juices into a large non-stick pan or wok over a medium heat. Add the garlic and cook for 1–2 minutes until softened. Next, add the smoked paprika and stir to combine until the garlic is coated in the spice. Squeeze in the lemon juice, (catch the pips!) to add the zingy element. Cook until most of the juice evaporates.

Add the spinach (you may need to add it in two batches to fit) and cook until it has completely wilted. The spinach will release its own moisture, so allow the liquid from the wilted spinach to cook out) before adding the cream, soured cream, Parmesan and thyme leaves. Increase the heat and stir regularly for several minutes until you have a full-flavoured, thick, creamed spinach. This may take some time, so be patient. Season with a little salt and white pepper.

Divide the creamed spinach between 4 plates and serve the crispy chicken thighs over the top. Season with salt flakes and freshly ground black pepper if needed. Scatter over some more fresh thyme leaves if you have any more kicking about.

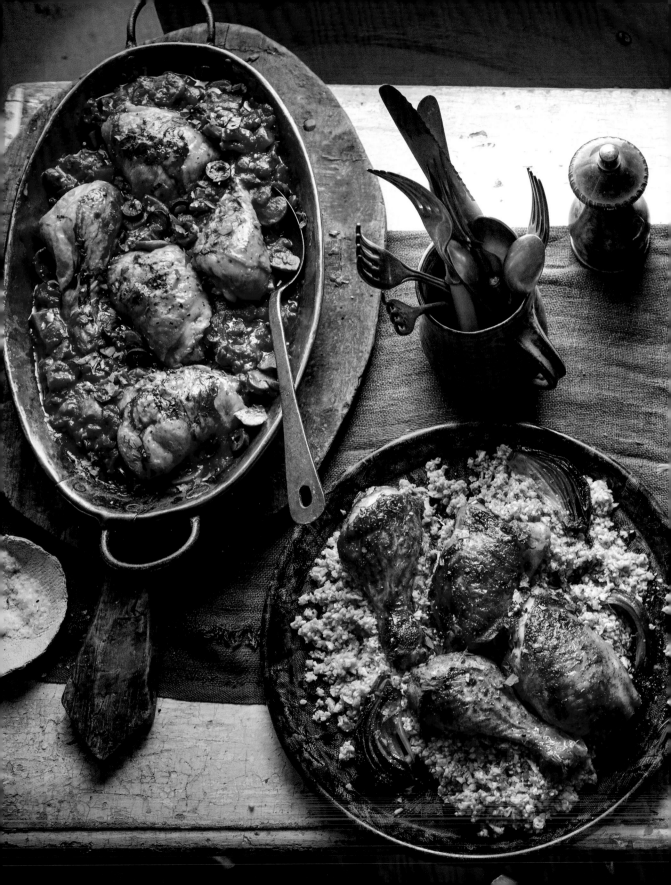

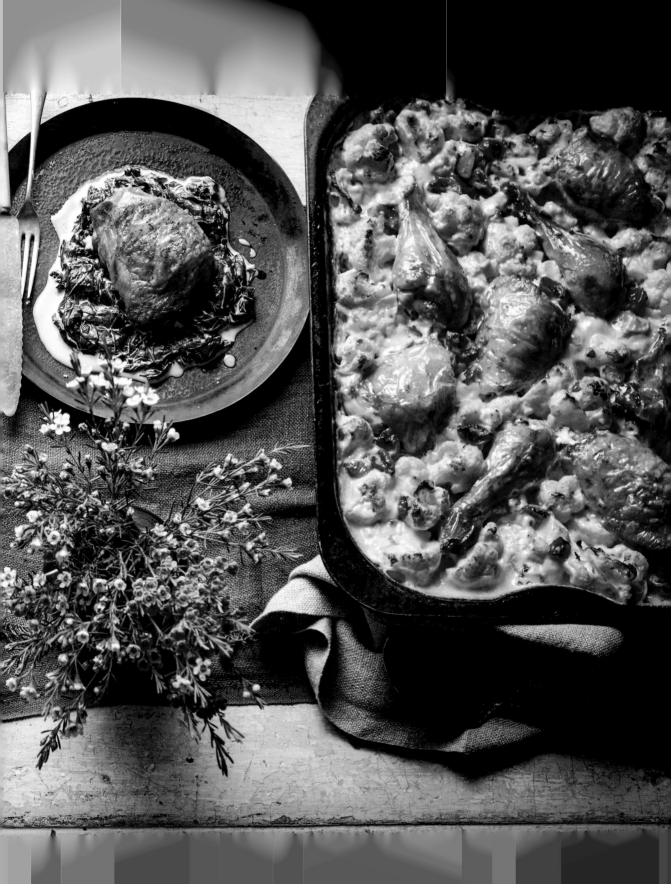

Chicken Cacciatore

I am not sure why it took me so long to include a simple cacciatore in one of my books! The flavours are deep, familiar and so, so satisfying. The slow cooking of the chicken means the meat falls off the bones – so please check for bones when tucking in! You can use thighs or drumsticks here, or, indeed, a combination of both, as long as they are cooked through safely. Lovely served over the Creamy Cauliflower Rice (page 29, excluded in these macros). Either parsley or basil will make a wonderful, fresh garnish, but I personally use a little of each when I have both on hand. *Pictured on page 98.*

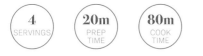

4 SERVINGS | **20m** PREP TIME | **80m** COOK TIME

CALORIES 483 | CARBS 8.2G | FAT 32G | PROTEIN 39G

1 tablespoon lard or ghee

8 chicken pieces (thighs and drumsticks), approx. 1.2kg (2lb 10oz) total weight

½ onion, finely chopped

3 garlic cloves, finely chopped

200g (7oz) mushrooms, sliced

1 teaspoon dried oregano

60ml (4 tablespoons) red wine

400g (14oz) can chopped tomatoes

1 tablespoon double-concentrated tomato purée

120ml (4fl oz) chicken stock

50g (1¾oz) pitted black olives, drained and sliced (drained weight)

small handful of fresh flat-leaf parsley or basil leaves

finely grated zest of 1 lemon

salt flakes, salt and freshly ground black pepper

Heat the lard or ghee in your largest non-stick pan or wok over a high heat while you season the chicken pieces all over with a little salt. Add the chicken (skin-side down) to the pan and brown for 2–3 minutes or until the skins are golden and crispy. Turn them over and cook the underside for 1 minute until it gets a little colour. Use tongs to remove the chicken pieces and set aside on a large platter, skin-side up.

You should still have plenty of fat in the pan. Reduce the heat to medium and add the onion, cooking for 10–11 minutes until softened. Add the garlic, and cook, stirring regularly, for 1–2 minutes until the onion begins to caramelise and the garlic softens. Increase the heat to high and add the mushrooms and dried oregano. Continue to cook, stirring, until the mushrooms release all their moisture and start to caramelise. Pour in the red wine, which will deglaze the pan. Once all the wine has evaporated, add the chopped tomatoes, tomato purée and chicken stock. Bring to the boil, then reduce to a simmer and stir in the olives. Now return the chicken pieces to the pan, along with any resting juices from the platter, nestling the chicken in amongst the mixture in an even layer. Cover with a lid and leave over a low–medium heat to simmer for 1 hour, removing the lid for the last 30 minutes.

By now, the sauce will have thickened and the chicken should be succulent, but safely cooked through. If in doubt, use a thermometer probed into the thickest part of the thigh: it should read 72°C (161°F).

Season with salt flakes and freshly ground black pepper, and garnish with parsley or basil and the lemon zest just before serving. Enjoy over your favourite base, such as cauliflower mash or buttered courgetti.

Chicken, Cauli & Tomato Basil Bake

This bake was inspired by a combination of three separate dishes I feature on my blog, Fats of Life® (www.fatsoflife.co.uk) and the result is simply superb! It's like a cauliflower cheese bake met some beautifully cooked chicken pieces, then they got married and asked basil to perform the ceremony! The tomato adds a little sweetness to cut through the rich flavours, and the basil (an essential component) finishes it all off beautifully. You will love it – and not only because it is so easy! *Pictured on page 99.*

4 SERVINGS | **15m** PREP TIME | **50m** COOK TIME

CALORIES 980 | CARBS 8.7G | FAT 83G | PROTEIN 48G

8 chicken pieces (thighs and drumsticks), approx. 1.2kg (2lb 10oz) total weight

500g (1lb 2oz) cauliflower florets

1 teaspoon unsalted butter

2 garlic cloves, finely chopped

380ml (12¾fl oz) double cream

50g (1¾oz) soured cream

60g (2¼oz) Parmesan or Pecorino cheese, finely grated

4 fresh thyme sprigs, leaves picked

300g (10½oz) cherry tomatoes, quartered

generous handful of fresh basil leaves, thinly sliced (see Tip)

salt flakes, salt, ground white pepper and freshly ground black pepper

Basil (a herb that should be stored at room temperature) is best sliced just before garnishing and serving to prevent it blackening.

Preheat the oven to 200°C/180°C fan/400°F/gas mark 6.

Place the chicken, skin-side up, in a large, deep roasting dish and bake for 20 minutes.

Meanwhile, bring a large pan of salted water to the boil. Add the cauliflower and cook for 13–14 minutes until tender. Drain well in a colander and leave to steam dry. This is essential to avoid a watery bake.

Remove the chicken from the oven and set aside (skin-side up) on a plate. Pour all the fat and rendered juices from the roasting dish into a large non-stick pan or wok over a medium heat. Add the butter and garlic and cook for 1–2 minutes until the garlic softens. Add the cream, soured cream, Parmesan and thyme leaves and bring to a simmer, then add the drained cauliflower to the pan, along with the tomatoes. Cook for 1–2 minutes, seasoning with a little white pepper and stirring well, then tip the whole lot back into the original roasting dish.

Return the chicken pieces to the dish, nestling them into the cauliflower mixture. Return to the oven for 20 minutes to bake the cream and cook the chicken through sufficiently.

Season with salt flakes and freshly ground black pepper and garnish with the all-important basil leaves just before serving.

Faux Truffle Pesto

This faux truffle pesto is made using a combination of mushrooms, black olives and the all-important truffle-infused oil. This delicious flavoured oil will last you a long time, as truffle has such a powerful (and luxurious) taste that it's likely you will only reach for it on special occasions. This pesto is ideal for mushroom-lovers and fans of the 'fifth taste', umami, because it is packed with both. A batch of this pesto serves four people (at 60g/2¼oz per serving), and this is what the macros indicate.

4 SERVINGS | **10m** PREP TIME | **30m** COOK TIME

CALORIES 190 | CARBS 2.3G | FAT 20G | PROTEIN 2.5G

40g (1½oz) pitted black olives, drained and thinly sliced (drained weight)

10g (¼oz) unsalted butter

220g (7¾oz) mushrooms, finely chopped

2 garlic cloves, finely chopped

1 tablespoon finely grated Parmesan or Pecorino cheese

5 tablespoons truffle-infused olive oil

salt and freshly ground black pepper

Preheat the oven to 140°C/120°C fan/275°F/gas mark 1 and line a small baking tray with baking paper.

Spread out the sliced olives on the prepared tray and place in the oven for 25–30 minutes to completely dry out.

Meanwhile, melt the butter in a large non-stick frying pan or wok over a high heat and add the finely chopped mushrooms and garlic. Cook for 8–10 minutes until the mixture is completely free from moisture. As they cook, the mushrooms will release their own moisture, so this needs to be cooked out too in order for them to start caramelising. Stir regularly to prevent the garlic burning.

The mixture will be ready once the mushrooms are golden and the pan is free of moisture. Remove from the heat and allow to cool a little while you wait for the olives to finish their time in the oven.

Transfer the cooked mushrooms and dried olive slices into a mini food processor or food chopper. Add the Parmesan and blitz well. It's good practice to stop and scrape down the sides every now and then to ensure even blitzing. Add 2 tablespoons of the truffle-infused olive oil and blitz one last time.

Transfer the pesto to a bowl and stir through the remaining truffle-infused olive oil. Season generously with salt and freshly ground black pepper.

If you decide to make this ahead of time, you can keep it, covered, in the fridge for 2–3 days. However, you need to bring it back up to room temperature again before serving, or place it in a very low oven to gently warm up.

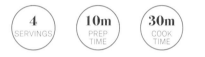

This pesto is delicious served over steak or stirred through your favourite low-carb noodles – but remember, the macros here are just for the pesto.

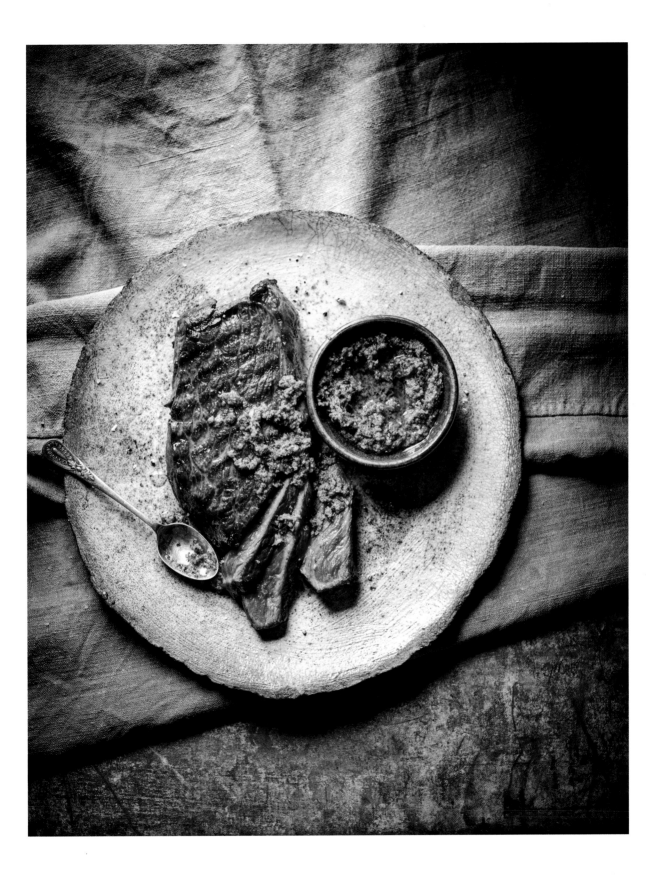

Steak & Egg Stir-fry

I used inexpensive frying steaks for this stir-fry, but you can use any steak that fits your budget. I also add eggs, so this will be a relatively high-protein meal (which is OK – even essential – for many people, depending on their physical activity). If you prefer a lower-protein meal, simply reduce the quantity of steak or eggs – but keep the rest of the ingredients in, because they are simply delicious when fried up like this! *Pictured here with Thai-style Red Beef Curry (see page 109).*

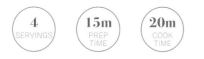

4 SERVINGS | **15m** PREP TIME | **20m** COOK TIME

CALORIES 367 | CARBS 4.8G | FAT 21G | PROTEIN 39G

400g (14oz) frying steaks, patted dry and sliced into thin strips

2 teaspoons ground ginger

2 tablespoons coconut oil

3 garlic cloves, finely chopped

1 lemongrass stalk, finely chopped (hard outer layer discarded)

2 red chillies, finely chopped, plus extra to garnish (optional)

300g (10½oz) mushrooms, sliced

juice of 1 lime

4 large eggs, whisked

2 tablespoon tamari (gluten-free soy sauce – see Tip on page 75)

1 tablespoon toasted sesame oil

2 spring onions, sliced

Place the steak strips in a bowl and scatter over the ginger. Toss well to evenly coat. The mixture will look quite dry, which is perfect.

Heat the coconut oil in a large non-stick pan or wok over a high heat. Working in batches, add the steak strips and fry for 1–2 minutes just until they are browned and caramelised on the outside. Remove from the pan using tongs and set aside on a plate while you fry the next batch. Doing this in batches avoids overcrowding the pan, which can result in the steak simmering as opposed to flash-frying which caramelises the pieces, resulting in better flavour.

Once you've fried and removed the final batch, there should still be plenty of fat remaining in the pan. If not, add a little more coconut oil. Reduce the heat to medium and add the garlic, lemongrass and chillies. Cook for 3–4 minutes, stirring regularly until they soften completely. Add the mushrooms and increase the heat to high until the mushrooms caramelise. Cook for 3–4 minutes, stirring continuously to prevent the garlic burning.

Squeeze in the lime juice and cook until there is no more moisture in the pan. Tip in the whisked eggs and stir well as they begin to scramble among the other elements. Once the eggs have scrambled, add the tamari, then return the steak strips to the pan.

Gently warm the whole lot through, drizzling over the sesame oil just before serving.

Garnish with plenty of sliced spring onions and red chillies (if using). Delicious as is, or enjoy over courgetti or your favourite low-carb noodles.

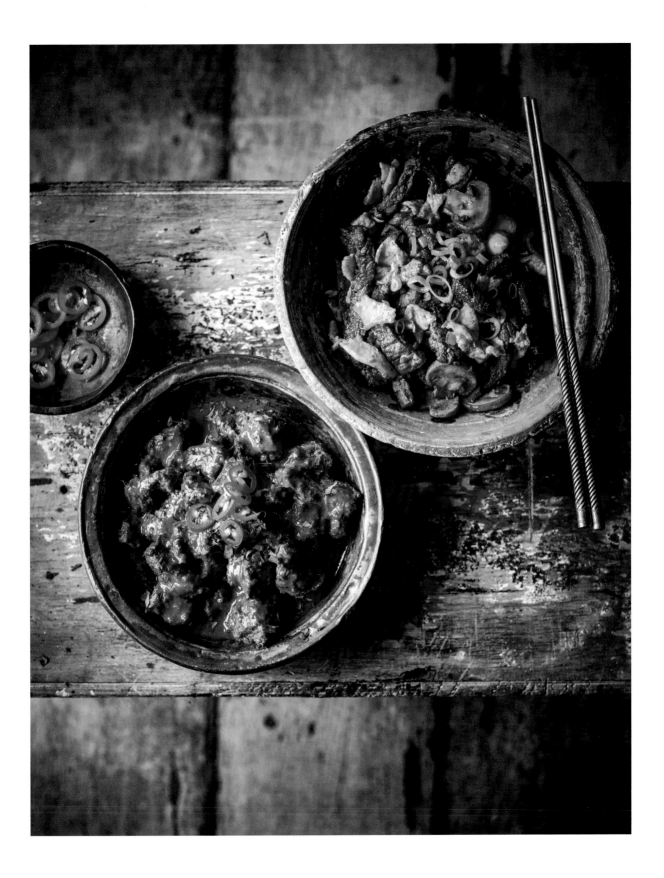

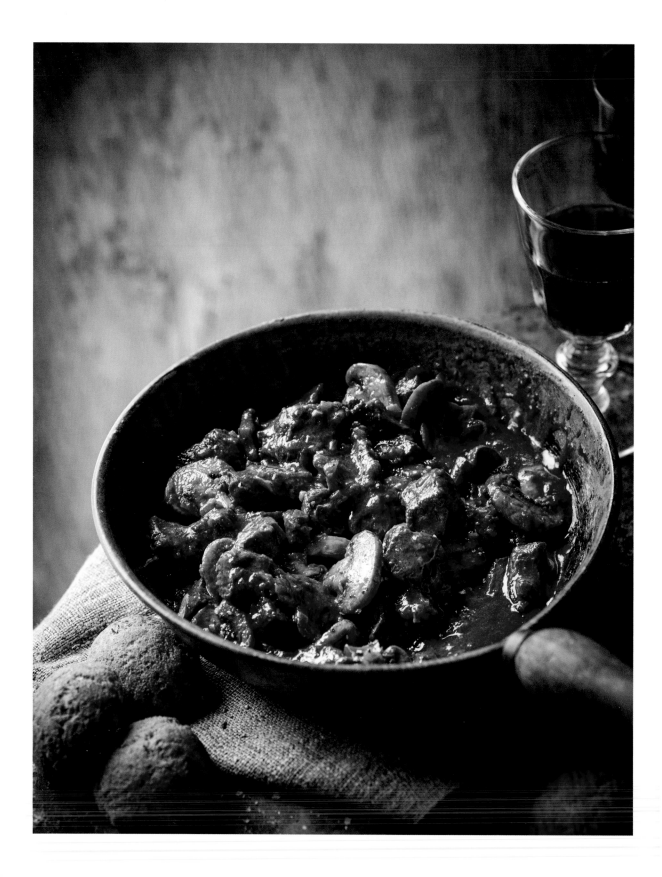

Poor Man's Bourguignon

with Mini Bread Rolls

A high-quality red wine is an important element in a classic Beef Bourguignon, but I personally don't pay too much attention to that, because any affordable red wine will still deliver a rich, deep flavour! I thicken the sauce with arrowroot powder, which does a great job in place of traditionally used cornflour. Best of all, though, are the miniature bread rolls (included in the macros). These rolls are best enjoyed warm, and are lovely buttered and served alongside the stew.

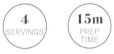

4 SERVINGS | **15m** PREP TIME | **3h** COOK TIME

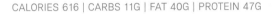

CALORIES 616 | CARBS 11G | FAT 40G | PROTEIN 47G

1 tablespoon lard or ghee

600g (1lb 5oz) stewing beef chunks, patted dry

2 tablespoons unsalted butter

½ onion, finely chopped

2 garlic cloves, finely chopped

200g (7oz) mushrooms, thickly sliced

½ teaspoon smoked paprika

3 fresh thyme sprigs, leaves picked

60ml (4 tablespoons) red wine

500ml (18fl oz) beef stock

2 tablespoons double-concentrated tomato purée

1 tablespoon arrowroot powder (or use 1 x 8g/¼oz sachet)

2 tablespoons water

ingredients continued overleaf

Melt the lard or ghee in a large saucepan over a high heat. Working in batches, fry the beef pieces for 2–3 minutes until they are golden on all sides. Set each batch aside in a large bowl when it's done. It's best to do this in batches so as not to overcrowd the pan, which would result in the beef simmering as opposed to browning.

Once all the beef is cooked and set aside, I like to switch to using butter! Melt 1 tablespoon of the butter in the same pan, reducing the heat to medium. Add the onion and fry for 10–11 minutes until softened. Add the garlic and continue to cook for 1–2 minutes until this too has softened. Add the remaining tablespoon of butter and stir in the mushrooms, smoked paprika and thyme. Increase the heat to high and stir continuously for 7–10 minutes until the mushrooms have released all their moisture and are starting to caramelise. Be careful not to burn the garlic.

Add the red wine to deglaze the pan and cook until the wine reduces to a thick, syrupy mixture. Pour in the beef stock – along with the tomato purée – and reduce the heat, bringing the mixture to a simmer. Return the beef chunks to the pan. Mix the arrowroot powder and water together in a small bowl or ramekin and add to the mixture. Cover with a cartouche (see page 30) and simmer over a low heat for 2 hours until the stew has a lovely thick consistency. You may want to remove the cartouche towards the end if the sauce has not reduced and thickened to your liking.

Meanwhile, make the mini bread rolls. Preheat the oven to 200°C/180°C fan/400°F/gas mark 6 and line a baking tray with baking paper.

✳ *continued overleaf*

Poor Man's Bourguignon

with Mini Bread Rolls
(continued)

For the mini bread rolls

60ml (4 tablespoons) warm water

1 teaspoon inulin powder

10g (¼oz) dried active yeast

4 large eggs, whisked

1 tablespoon olive oil

60g (2¼oz) unsalted butter, melted

50g (1¾oz) coconut flour

¾ teaspoon baking powder

1 teaspoon salt

½ teaspoon garlic powder

3–4 fresh thyme sprigs, leaves picked

25g (1oz) psyllium husk powder

*

If you prefer to use almond flour in the mini bread rolls, replace the coconut flour with 100g (3½oz) almond flour. However, an almond flour mixture will not thicken enough to 'roll' into little balls because it doesn't absorb moisture like coconut flour does. In that case, just spoon 12 little, even-sized mounds onto the baking tray.

Pour the warm water into a small bowl or ramekin. Stir in the inulin powder to dissolve. Leave the water to cool until tepid (hot water will kill the yeast). Scatter the yeast over the top and stir well to combine. Set aside for 15 minutes until the surface is frothy and the mixture has grown significantly in size.

In a second, medium-sized bowl, whisk together the eggs and olive oil. Once the melted butter has cooled a little, whisk this in, too. In a third, large bowl, combine the coconut flour, baking powder, salt, garlic powder and thyme leaves, ensuring there are no lumps.

Once the yeast mixture has visibly activated, tip the whole lot into the egg mixture and whisk well to combine. Next, pour this wet mixture into the bowl with the coconut flour mixture and whisk vigorously to form a smooth batter. Add the psyllium husk powder, then immediately whisk vigorously – it will get to work very quickly thickening the mixture. Once combined, set the bowl aside for 2 minutes to stiffen and thicken further.

Use a small spoon to divide the mixture into 12 even-sized portions. They will be soft, but should still be easy to roll into little balls. Place the balls on the prepared tray and bake on the lowest rack for 8 minutes, then reduce the oven temperature to 170°C/150°C fan/340°F/gas mark 3½ and bake for another 10–12 minutes. (Halfway through baking, I always quickly rotate my tray and then lay a sheet of foil over the rolls to prevent the tops darkening too much.)

Serve the finished stew with the little bread rolls, which you can halve and butter before dipping in! This would also be lovely over some cauliflower mash if your macros allow for it.

Thai-style Red Beef Curry

The flavours of this curry are fresh and hearty, and bring back fond memories of some of the travelling Mark and I have done over the years. I've used inexpensive stewing beef in this recipe: it needs to be cooked low and slow to become tender. You could make this curry in a slow-cooker if you prefer – you just need to remove the lid for the last 45 minutes so the sauce can reduce and thicken. *Pictured on page 105.*

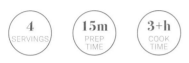

4 SERVINGS | **15m** PREP TIME | **3+h** COOK TIME

CALORIES 591 | CARBS 6.2G | FAT 43G | PROTEIN 45G

800g (1lb 12oz) stewing beef chunks, patted dry

1 teaspoon ground coriander

1 teaspoon garlic powder

½ teaspoon ground turmeric

40g (1½oz) coconut oil

400g (14oz) can full-fat coconut milk

salt

handful of fresh coriander leaves, finely chopped

sliced red chillies, to serve (optional)

For the curry paste

50g (1¾oz) red chillies (approx. 3–4), deseeded and roughly chopped

1 lemongrass stalk, roughly chopped (hard outer layer discarded)

½ red onion, roughly chopped

4 garlic cloves, roughly chopped

25g (1oz) fresh root ginger, peeled and roughly chopped

juice of 1 lime

½ teaspoon ground coriander

pinch of ground cinnamon

2 tablespoons coconut oil, melted

To make the curry paste, place all the ingredients in a mini food processor or food chopper. Blitz until completely smooth, stopping to scrape down the sides a few times to ensure a smooth mixture. I often find that adding a tablespoon or two of hot water will assist in bringing the mixture together. Once done, set aside.

Tip the beef into a large bowl and scatter over the ground coriander, garlic powder and turmeric. Toss well to evenly coat. Cook in 4–5 batches for best results. For each batch, heat 1 teaspoon of coconut oil in a large, deep non-stick saucepan or wok over a high heat and fry some of the beef cubes for 1–2 minutes until golden on all sides. Remove using a slotted spoon and set aside in a bowl, then repeat with the rest.

Once you have fried and set aside all the beef, place the same pan or wok over a low–medium heat and add the curry paste. Cook for 1–2 minutes, stirring well. The lime juice in the curry paste will automatically deglaze the pan, lifting up any bits of meat that may have stuck (and adding additional flavour!). Pour in the coconut milk and increase the heat, bringing the mixture to the boil.

Once boiling, reduce the heat to a low simmer. Return the beef to the pan (along with any resting juices from the bowl) and leave on this low heat, partially covered, for 2½–3 hours, stirring occasionally, until the sauce has reduced down and the meat is tender. You may want to remove the lid completely during the last 20–30 minutes if the sauce has not reduced and thickened enough to your liking.

Season with salt if needed and serve scattered with chopped coriander and sliced red chillies, if using. This is delicious over buttered courgetti or your favourite low-carb noodles.

Ginger Pork Stir-fry

If you feel the need to cut back a little on fat (this often happens to me in summer months, when I feel like a lighter meal), you can always opt for pork tenderloin (also called fillet). Pork is an inexpensive meat and often referred to as the 'other' white meat because it is quite lean. Here, I've paired it with a handful of other ingredients you probably already have in your keto arsenal to make a delicious stir-fry that boasts just a tiny hint of sweetness. If you don't have sugar-free syrup, use a teaspoon or two of powdered erythritol.

4 SERVINGS | **15m** PREP TIME | **20m** COOK TIME

CALORIES 332 | CARBS 5.8G | FAT 14G | PROTEIN 44G

300g (10½oz) broccoli florets, trimmed into smaller pieces

500g (1lb 2oz) pork tenderloin, thinly sliced or chopped small (see Tip)

1 tablespoon ground ginger

2 tablespoons coconut oil

3 garlic cloves, finely chopped

30g (1oz) fresh root ginger, peeled and finely chopped

1 red chilli, finely sliced

6 spring onions, white parts thickly sliced, green ends thinly sliced and kept separate

1 tablespoon rice wine vinegar

1 tablespoon tamari (gluten-free soy sauce)

1 teaspoon sugar-free syrup

1 tablespoon toasted sesame oil

1 teaspoon sesame seeds

salt and freshly ground black pepper

*

You can use chicken in place of pork if you want, but it will need a little longer to safely cook through.

Bring a large pan of salted water to the boil and cook the broccoli for 3–4 minutes until tender. Drain well in a colander and leave to steam dry.

Pat the pork strips dry with a paper towel, then place in a large bowl and add the ground ginger. Season generously with salt and pepper, and toss well until all the pork is evenly coated. It will look quite dry, which is perfect.

Heat half the coconut oil in a large non-stick frying pan or wok over a high heat. Add the pork strips and fry for 2–3 minutes until golden and caramelised. This is best done in batches. Set aside in a bowl.

Reduce the heat to low and add the remaining coconut oil to the same pan. Add the garlic, ginger and chilli and cook, stirring regularly, for 2–3 minutes until softened. Increase the heat and add the rice wine vinegar, which will almost immediately cook out as it deglazes the pan.

Next, return the pork to the pan, along with the cooked broccoli and white parts of the spring onion. Increase the heat to medium–high and add the tamari and sugar-free syrup, stirring well for another minute or two to warm the whole lot through. Don't leave it on the heat for too long, as you don't want to dry out the pork.

Just before serving, drizzle over the sesame oil and scatter over the sesame seeds. Garnish with the green ends of the spring onions.

This is delicious as is, or can be enjoyed over courgetti, or your favourite low-carb noodles.

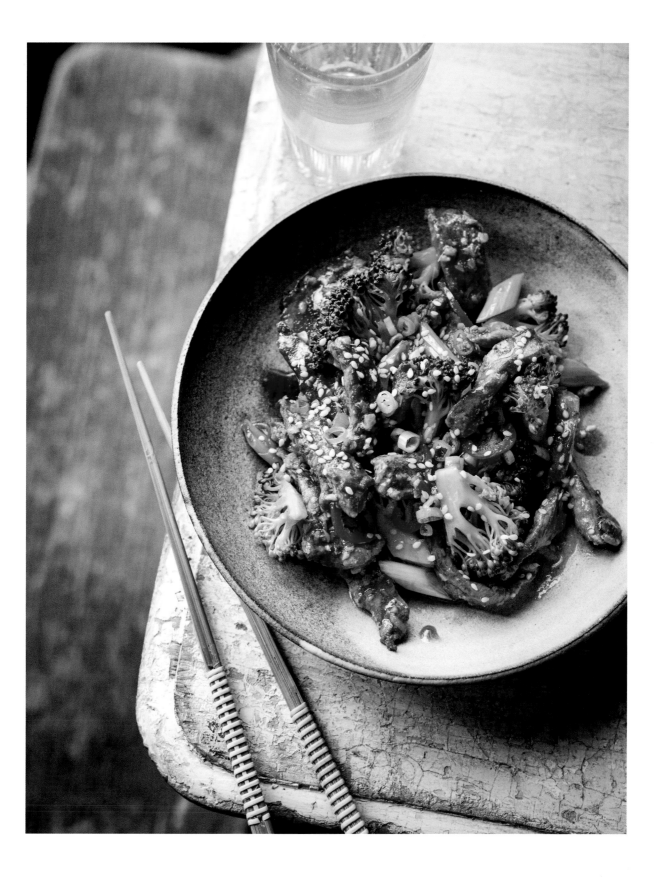

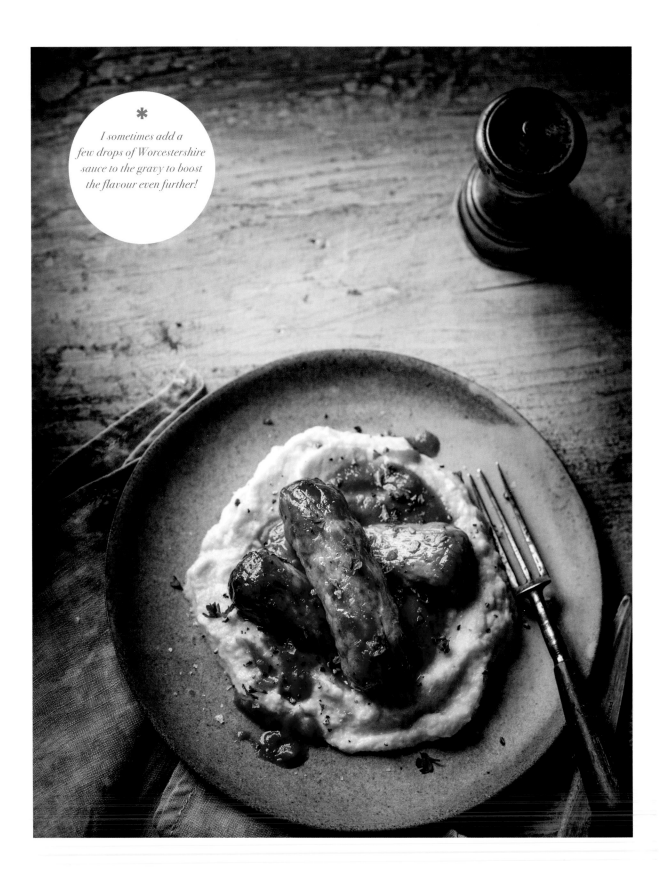

*

I sometimes add a few drops of Worcestershire sauce to the gravy to boost the flavour even further!

Bangers & Mash!

This hearty meal took me a long time to get Just Right. I used pork sausages here (aim for 97 per cent pork and gluten-free), served over a creamy cauliflower mash. However, the best part is the sharp but hearty keto gravy, to which I have added a tomato for sweetness and tang. This is a winner in our home – and all this from the humble porkie!

4 SERVINGS

25m PREP TIME

1h COOK TIME

8 gluten-free pork sausages

450g (1lb) cauliflower, chopped into small, even-sized pieces

45g (1½oz) full-fat cream cheese

40g (1½oz) unsalted butter

½ onion, thinly sliced

2 garlic cloves, finely chopped

1 tomato, chopped

200ml (7fl oz) chicken stock

handful of fresh flat-leaf parsley leaves, finely chopped

salt flakes, salt, ground white pepper and freshly ground black pepper

Gluten-free pork sausages are low in carbs, but they are considered 'dirty' keto because they contain a little added starch. This has never bothered me, because... well, porkies ROCK!

CALORIES 578 | CARBS 10G | FAT 46G | PROTEIN 28G

Preheat the oven to 200°C/180°C fan/400°F/gas mark 6 and grease a roasting dish.

Place the sausages in the prepared roasting dish and cook in the oven for 25 minutes until golden and cooked through. Remove and set aside to keep warm, but do not discard any rendered fat and juices that may be in the roasting dish.

Meanwhile, bring a large saucepan of salted water to the boil. Add the cauliflower and cook until completely softened; this can take up to 15 minutes. A good way to test is to pierce a floret with a fork: it should immediately slide off. Drain well in a colander and allow to steam off completely, this prevents a watery mash.

Wipe the saucepan dry and return the cauliflower to the pan. Add the cream cheese and three-quarters of the butter. Use a potato masher to mash well. Season with salt and white pepper and set aside to keep warm.

Meanwhile, make the gravy. Heat the remaining butter in a medium-sized saucepan over a medium heat. Add the onion and cook for 10–11 minutes until softened. Tip in the garlic and chopped tomato, and cook for 5–6 minutes until the garlic softens, the tomato breaks down and the whole lot becomes an orange mush! Pour in the stock, along with any fat and juices scraped from the porkies' roasting pan. Remove from the heat and use a hand blender to blitz until smooth. Return to the heat and simmer over a medium heat until the sauce is thick enough to coat the back of the spoon – this will take about 20–25 minutes.

Serve the sausages over the mash and pour over the gravy. Scatter over the chopped parsley and season with salt flakes and freshly ground black pepper.

'Choucroute'
with Sausage & Bacon

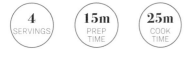

(4) SERVINGS (15m) PREP TIME (35m) COOK TIME

4 gluten-free pork sausages

40g (1½oz) Garlic-infused Browned Butter
(page 18)

100g (3½oz) smoked bacon lardons

pinch of ground allspice

250g (9oz) Savoy cabbage, sliced or shredded

1 tablespoon apple cider vinegar

60ml (4 tablespoons) water

1 tablespoon finely grated Parmesan cheese

small handful of fresh flat-leaf parsley leaves,
finely chopped

freshly ground black pepper

This isn't really a choucroute, but it boasts the same acidic flavours of vinegar and cooked cabbage, which pair wonderfully with the chunks of cooked pork sausages and smoked bacon lardons. If you can't get bacon lardons, just use chopped smoked streaky bacon.

CALORIES 406 | CARBS 5.2G | FAT 34G | PROTEIN 18G

Preheat the oven to 200°C/180°C fan/400°F/gas mark 6 and grease a roasting tray. Spread the pork sausages out on the prepared tray and roast for 25 minutes, then remove and set aside to cool for 10 minutes before chopping into bite-sized pieces.

Melt the garlic butter in a large non-stick pan or wok over a medium heat. Add the bacon lardons and cook for 6–8 minutes, then add the allspice, followed by the cabbage. Stir well, increasing the heat to high. Pour in the vinegar and water and cook, stirring, for 3–4 minutes until the cabbage is tender and there is no excess moisture in the pan. Stir through the sausages and Parmesan and season with black pepper. Once warmed through, serve with a scattering of chopped parsley.

'Dirty Rice'
with Bacon & Mushrooms

(4) SERVINGS (15m) PREP TIME (25m) COOK TIME

300g (10½oz) cauliflower florets, blitzed
into 'rice'

4 large eggs

50g (1¾oz) unsalted butter

250g (9oz) smoked streaky bacon, finely chopped

3 garlic cloves, finely chopped

300g (10½oz) mushrooms, sliced

6 spring onions, thinly sliced

juice of ½ lemon

2 teaspoons tamari (gluten-free soy sauce)

freshly ground black pepper

This dish was inspired by my Aunty Sandy's famous rice salad, which she brings to family gatherings in South Africa. I have missed many since moving to the UK, but I created this version to help with my nostalgia, with added eggs to increase protein.

CALORIES 372 | CARBS 5.9G | FAT 31G | PROTEIN 21G

Place the cauliflower 'rice' in a large, wide-bottomed microwave-safe bowl and microwave on high for 6 minutes. Set aside. Meanwhile, boil or poach the eggs to your liking and set aside to keep warm.

Melt the butter in a large non-stick pan over a medium heat. Add the bacon and garlic and cook for 9–10 minutes until the bacon releases all its juices and the garlic softens. Add the mushrooms and half the spring onions. Increase the heat to high and cook for 7–8 minutes until the mushrooms start to caramelise, stirring regularly. Add the lemon juice and cauliflower 'rice' and cook for 2–3 minutes, then add the tamari and stir well to combine. Season very generously with freshly ground black pepper, then scatter over the remaining spring onions and serve with the eggs on top!

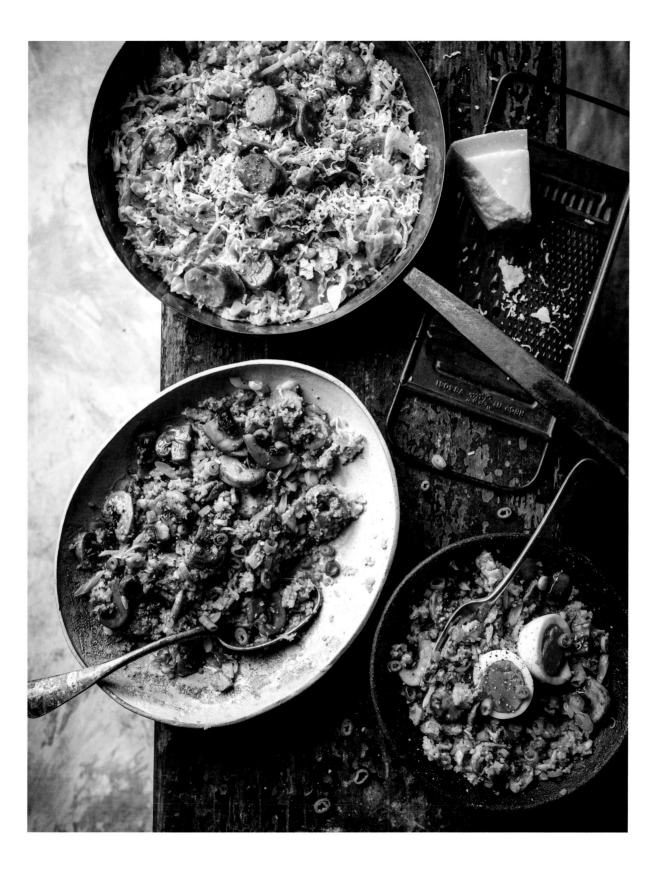

Sausage & Broccoli Bake

with Parmesan & Lemon

Mark turned his nose up a little when I told him what I was trying the first night I threw this meal together. 'Lemon and sausages?' he asked, unconvinced. Well, he loved it, and now regularly requests this hearty dish, which I have tweaked and perfected over time. It ticks all the boxes: quick, easy, delicious. What more could you ask for, come dinner time?

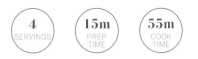

4 SERVINGS   **15m** PREP TIME   **55m** COOK TIME

CALORIES 821 | CARBS 9G | FAT 75G | PROTEIN 28G

8 gluten-free pork sausages

1 teaspoon unsalted butter

2 garlic cloves, finely chopped

300ml (10fl oz) double cream

2 tablespoons grated Parmesan or Pecorino cheese

400g (14oz) broccoli, trimmed into equal-sized florets

finely grated zest of 1 lemon

salt flakes, salt, ground white pepper and freshly ground black pepper

Preheat the oven to 200°C/180°C fan/400°F/gas mark 6 and lightly grease a deep 25–30cm (10–12in) roasting dish.

Spread out the sausages on the prepared roasting dish and bake for 25 minutes, then remove the sausages from the dish and set aside for now. Do not turn the oven off, and keep the roasting dish handy.

Heat the butter in a large non-stick pan or wok over a medium heat. If there are any juices and rendered fat from the sausages in the roasting dish, add that too. Add the garlic and gently cook for 1–2 minutes until softened. Add the cream and 1 tablespoon of the Parmesan and warm the mixture through for 3–4 minutes, reducing the cream a little. Season with salt and ground white pepper.

Meanwhile, boil the broccoli in a large pan of salted water for 3–4 minutes until tender. Drain well in a colander and allow to steam off a little before adding to the creamy mixture in the pan. Pour the whole lot into the previously used roasting dish in a relatively even layer.

The sausages will have cooled a little by now. Slice them in half diagonally and add them to the roasting dish, nestling them in among the creamy broccoli. Bake for 20–25 minutes to allow the cream to cook down to a luxurious flavour!

To serve, scatter over the remaining Parmesan, along with the all-important lemon zest. Season with salt flakes (if needed) and plenty of freshly ground black pepper.

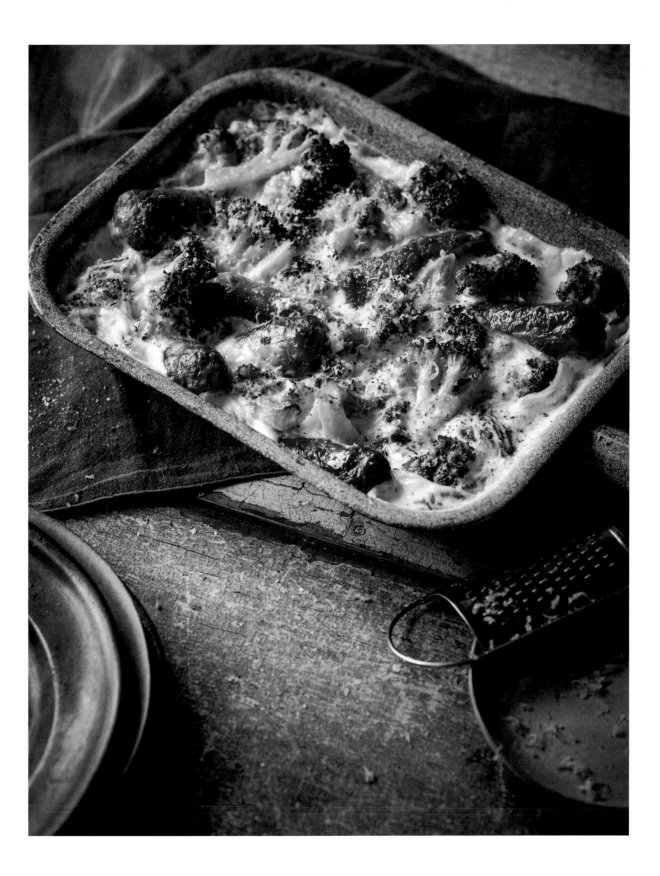

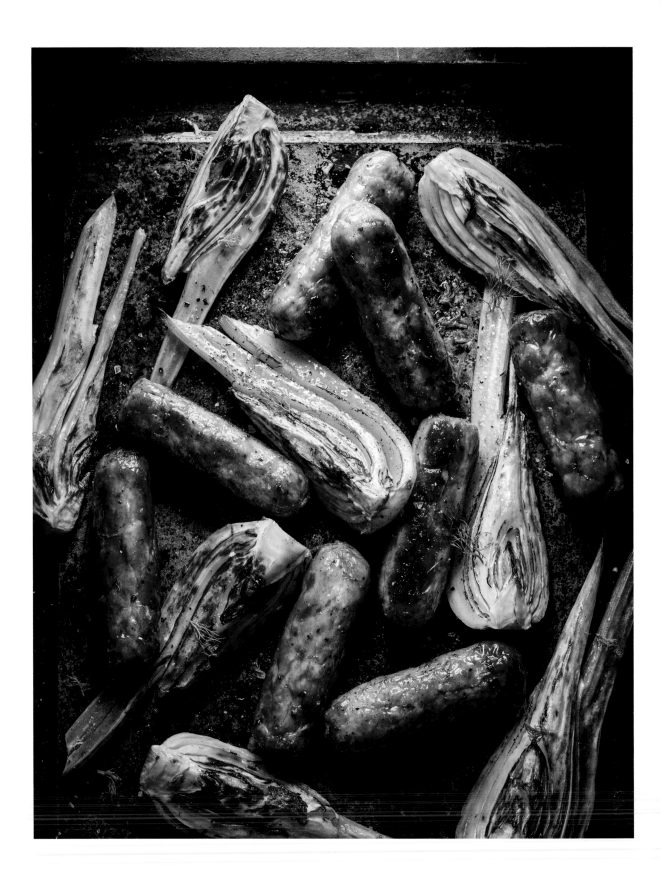

Sausages

with Roasted Fennel

In this beautiful, tasty one-tray dish, fragrant roasted fennel bulbs complement simple store-bought porkies. I try and eat a wide variety of low-carb vegetables because they all come with their own unique micro-nutrients (vitamins and minerals), and I want to encourage you to do the same on your keto journey. If you find this dish isn't filling enough for you, enjoy it with some cauliflower mash– and there is no judgement here if you want to add more sausages!

4 SERVINGS | **5m** PREP TIME | **25m** COOK TIME

CALORIES 456 | CARBS 6.1G | FAT 37G | PROTEIN 23G

2 large fennel bulbs, trimmed and quartered (see Tip), fronds reserved for garnish

8 gluten-free pork sausages

1 tablespoon olive oil

½ teaspoon garlic powder

salt flakes and freshly ground black pepper

Preheat the oven to 220°C/200°C fan/425°F/gas mark 7 and grease a large baking tray.

Place the fennel pieces and sausages in a bowl. Add the olive oil and garlic powder and gently toss the whole lot to evenly coat. (Work gently, as you don't want the fennel falling apart.)

Spread the whole lot out on the prepared baking tray and bake for 25 minutes. I always rotate the tray halfway through to ensure even cooking, and take this opportunity to turn over all the pieces using tongs.

Serve scattered with salt flakes and freshly ground black pepper. Sprinkle over the reserved fennel fronds for a fresh, pretty finish!

✳

Cut the fennel into quarters lengthways through the root end to ensure all the pieces remain intact.

Rosemary Belly Bites

with Cheesy Tomato Mash

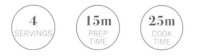

4 SERVINGS | 15m PREP TIME | 25m COOK TIME

These bite-sized pieces of pork belly are served over a delicious tomato cauli-mash that really steals the show in this easy dish. There is some additional work in making a garlic-infused butter and taking the time to finely chop rosemary needles, but I promise you it is worth the effort.

CALORIES 702 | CARBS 5.9G | FAT 53G | PROTEIN 49G

800g (1lb 12oz) pork belly slices, cut into chunks

3–4 rosemary sprigs, needles picked and finely chopped

500g (1lb 2oz) cauliflower florets, chopped into small, even-sized pieces

2 tomatoes, finely chopped

20g (¾oz) Garlic-infused Browned Butter (page 18), melted

75g (2¾oz) Gruyère cheese, finely grated

salt and freshly ground black pepper

Preheat the oven to 220°C/200°C fan/425°F/gas mark 7.

Lightly season the pork belly chunks and spread out on a baking tray. Cook in the oven for 24–25 minutes, then scatter over three-quarters of the finely chopped rosemary, stir well and set aside to keep warm.

Meanwhile, in a large saucepan of salted boiling water, cook the cauliflower for 18–20 minutes. Drain well, then return to the same pan (wiped dry) and use a potato masher to mash. Fold in the tomatoes, garlic butter and the remaining rosemary. Warm through for 2–3 minutes, adding the grated cheese in the last minute. Serve the pork belly pieces over the mash, seasoned with salt and pepper.

Chinese Pork Belly

with Sesame Avo Slaw

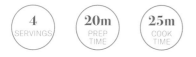

4 SERVINGS | 20m PREP TIME | 25m COOK TIME

This is a simple and tasty way to prepare pork belly slices, and the result is superb – especially when accompanied by this delicious cabbage and avocado slaw. We regularly have this dish, and it's one of my favourites in this book!

CALORIES 1051 | CARBS 4G | FAT 91G | PROTEIN 52G

1kg (2lb 4oz) pork belly slices

2 tablespoons Chinese five-spice

2 teaspoons tamari (gluten-free soy sauce)

200g (7oz) Savoy cabbage, thinly sliced

120g (4¼oz) mayonnaise

2 avocados, diced

4 spring onions, finely sliced

1 tablespoon toasted sesame oil

2 teaspoons sesame seeds

salt and freshly ground black pepper

Preheat the oven to 210°C/190°C fan/410°F/gas mark 6½ and line a baking tray with baking paper.

Place the pork belly slices in a large bowl and stir in the Chinese five-spice and tamari until evenly coated. Place on the prepared tray and bake on the middle rack for 24–25 minutes.

Meanwhile, combine the cabbage, mayonnaise, avocado and most of the spring onions in a bowl. Drizzle over the sesame oil and mix well.

Serve the pork with the slaw, seasoning both with salt and pepper. Scatter over the sesame seeds and remaining spring onions to garnish.

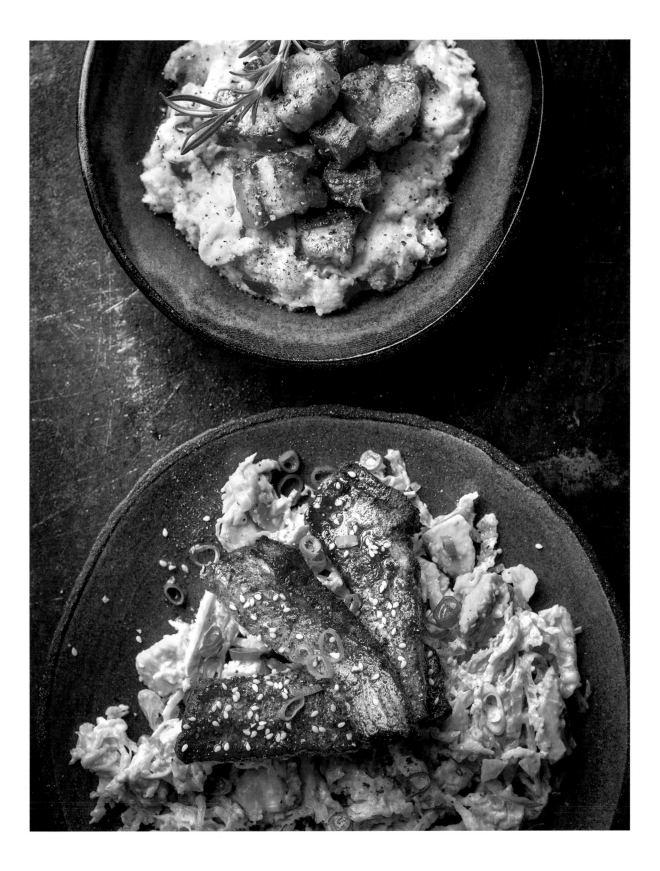

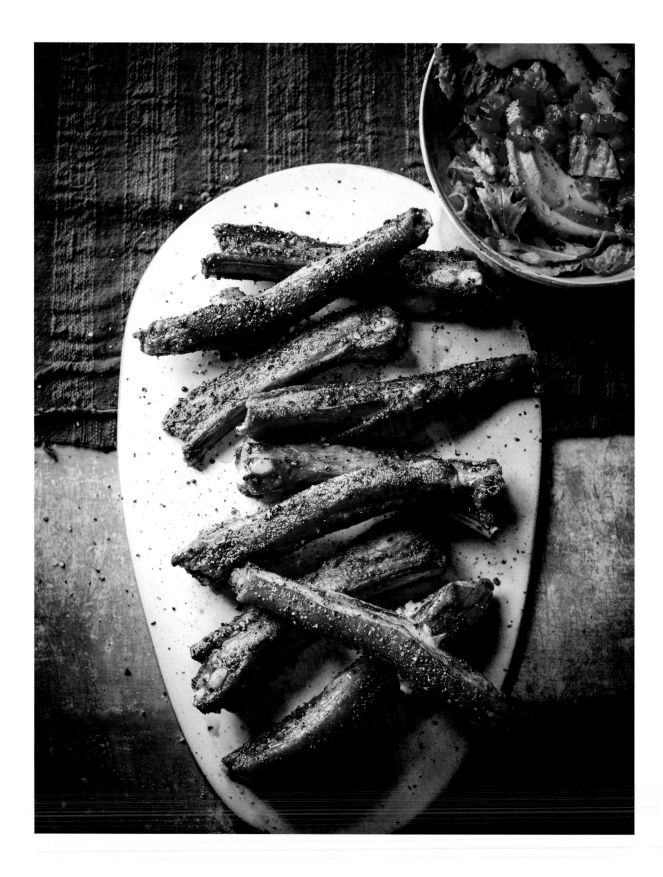

Peppered Lamb Riblets

with Our Favourite Salad

This decadent meal is one that we enjoy often at home. Lamb ribs are not available in all stores, but your butcher will source and sell them to you at a low cost because they are not a popular cut, it seems. Mark seasons these with generous cracks of black pepper prior to cooking, and they need little else apart from salt flakes after. Since lamb is gloriously fatty, we love it with this salad, where every ingredient is included for a reason. If you cannot source lamb ribs, do give the delicious salad a try anyway!

4 SERVINGS   **10m** PREP TIME   **30m** COOK TIME

CALORIES 1058 | CARBS 3.9G | FAT 91G | PROTEIN 53G

1kg (2lb 4oz) lamb ribs

salt, salt flakes and freshly ground black pepper

For the salad

100g (3½oz) romaine, cos or iceberg lettuce, roughly chopped

30g (1oz) wild rocket

handful of fresh flat-leaf parsley leaves, finely chopped

30g (1oz) finely grated Parmesan or Pecorino cheese

2 avocados, sliced

juice of 1 lemon

2 tomatoes, chopped

2 garlic cloves, crushed with a press

3 tablespoons olive oil

These can be made in your air-fryer too! While it may not have the South African gees (spirit) of a wood braai (barbecue), it will cook the lamb ribs to perfection.

Prepare your barbecue or preheat the oven to 210°C/190°C fan/410°F/gas mark 6½.

Remove the lamb ribs from their packaging and very generously season on all sides with freshly ground black pepper. If you're barbecuing, cook the ribs on the barbecue until the fat crisps up and the meat is cooked through. If you are making them in the oven, place them on a cooking rack set over a roasting tray and cook for 25–30 minutes until crispy and cooked through. Once cooked, season with salt flakes.

The salad can be prepared several hours ahead of time, but the elements should be kept separate for best results. Combine the lettuce, rocket, parsley and Parmesan in a large bowl and keep covered in the fridge. In a second, smaller bowl, toss the diced avocado with the generously squeezed fresh lemon juice. This not only brings an acidic element to the salad, but it also prevents the avocado blackening. Season with salt and pepper, then cover and leave in the fridge. In a third, small bowl, combine the tomatoes, crushed garlic and all the olive oil. Remember, the garlic is eaten raw in this salad, so please use a garlic press to crush the garlic to achieve the best texture and flavour. Season with salt and pepper, then cover and leave at room temperature. (I find chilled tomatoes lack flavour. Even in cases like this where I am prepping a tomato element for a salad, I keep it covered at room temperature where it will be perfectly fine for several hours.)

Combine all the salad elements in a large serving bowl just before serving. The lemon juice from the avocado bowl and the olive oil from the tomato bowl will combine to make up your dressing. It is unlikely the salad will need further seasoning.

Serve the delicious lamb ribs with the salad on the side. Too easy!

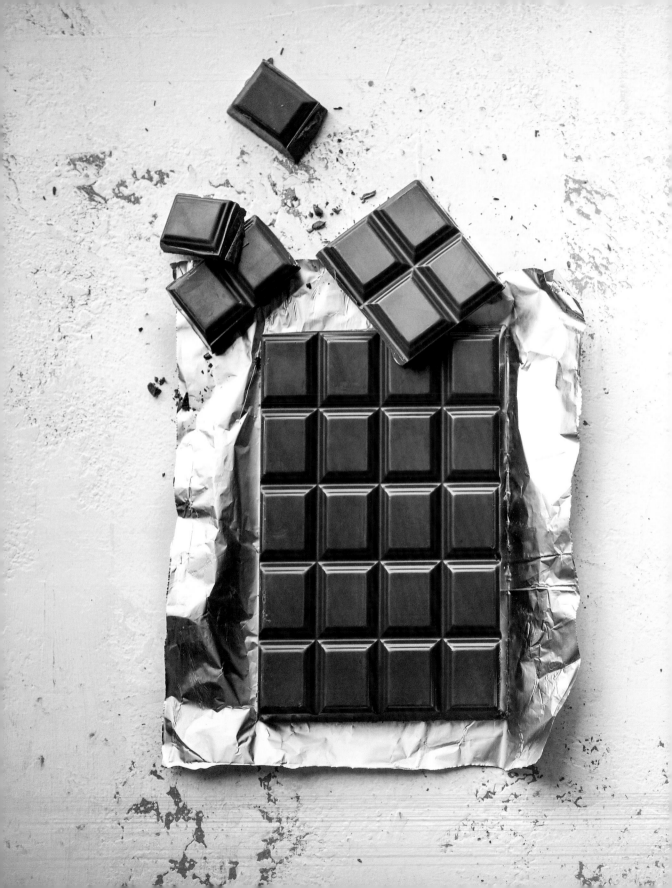

Sweet Treats

I have always enjoyed savoury food more than sweet, and I guess that is reflected in the length of the dessert chapters in my books, because I tend to keep them short and sweet (excuse the pun). This is also because I would rather encourage you to wean yourself off sweet things, as opposed to sticking a plaster on a sugar addiction. However, there are many people who find using a natural sweetener (like erythritol, which has no effect on blood sugar for most people) is a fantastic alternative that helps with making this transition.

This is not to say that I still don't churn out 'sweet' treats by the dozen – even now, so many years into our keto journey, Mark has not abandoned his sweet tooth, and probably never will. There is no judgement from me, though – in fact, I've relished the challenge of finding ways to satisfy his fondness for sweet things while staying true to the keto lifestyle!

My preferred natural sweetener has always been powdered erythritol, sifted before using. Some people find that erythritol leaves a 'cooling' effect on the palate, but adding just a few drops of liquid stevia can balance this out. I have added this as an option in the recipes where erythritol features in large quantities.

I hope you love this small collection of deliciously easy sweet treats!

Coconut Bites

with Chocolate Drizzle

These bite-sized morsels are dead easy to make. They are only 2.4g carbs per bite – and, if you choose not to decorate with the melted chocolate 'dip and drizzle', they will come in at only 1.1g carbs each (but who can resist adding chocolate?). These bites will store well in the fridge, covered, for 3–4 days, but are best enjoyed at room temperature with a cup of tea or coffee.

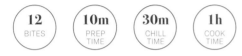

12 BITES	**10m** PREP TIME	**30m** CHILL TIME	**1h** COOK TIME

PER COCONUT BITE: CALORIES 94 | CARBS 2.4G | FAT 8G | PROTEIN 2.5G

85g (3oz) desiccated coconut

1 tablespoon coconut flour

pinch of salt

2 large egg whites

¼ teaspoon cream of tartar

½ teaspoon vanilla extract

2–3 drops liquid stevia (optional)

40g (1½oz) powdered erythritol, sifted

70g (2½oz) dark chocolate (85 per cent cocoa), broken into pieces

*

The uncooked mounds are fragile and can easily fall apart, so it's important to work carefully with them prior to baking, and just as they come out of the oven.

Combine the desiccated coconut, coconut flour and salt in a bowl.

In a second bowl, use a hand mixer to whip the egg whites and cream of tartar to stiff peaks. Add the vanilla, liquid stevia (if using) and erythritol and continue to whip until well combined. Tip the dry mix into this mixture and gently fold through to combine (try not to knock too much air out). Cover and place in the fridge to chill for 30 minutes.

Meanwhile, preheat the oven to 140°C/120°C fan/275°F/gas mark 1 and line 2 large baking trays with baking paper.

Divide the mixture into 12 ping-pong-ball-sized mounds. Use a dessert spoon and the palm of your hand to roll each one into a ball and gently place on one of the prepared trays (see Tip).

Bake on the lowest rack for 20 minutes, then reduce the oven temperature to 120°C/100°C/250°F/gas mark ½ and bake for an additional 20 minutes. I always rotate the tray every 10 minutes to ensure even colouring. Turn the oven off and leave the bites in the oven for further 20 minutes to finish cooking in the residual heat. You can place a sheet of foil on top if you don't want them to darken too much.

Carefully transfer each of the bites on to a cooling rack.

For the chocolate dip and drizzle, melt the chocolate in a small saucepan over a very low heat. Remove from the heat, and lightly dip the bottom of each cooled coconut bite into the chocolate. Place on the second lined tray with the chocolate-dipped part on the bottom. You will have enough melted chocolate left over to drizzle over the bites – this is easy to do using a fork. The chocolate will harden as it cools, so leave to set completely before enjoying .

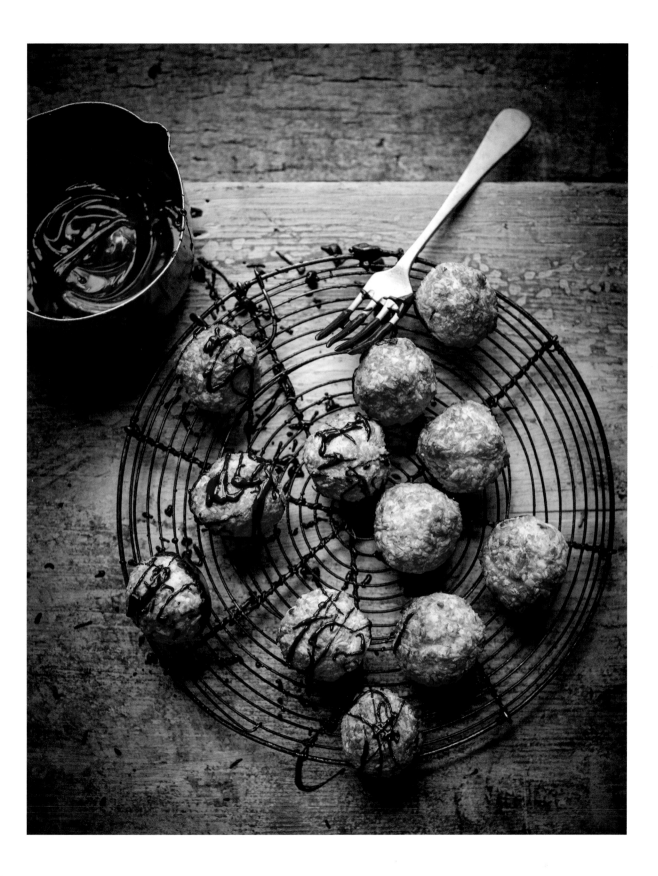

Warm Vanilla Pudding

with Homemade Custard

In many parts of the world, a 'pudding' is usually a sweet or savoury steamed item. In South Africa, however, 'pudding' refers to any dessert! This delicious, warm bake is inspired by a South African dessert called 'Malva pudding', but I excluded the elements that are not considered low-carb friendly. This is a sweet and comforting winter dessert, perfect for a crowd. It's finished with a super-sweet syrup, then generously drizzled with warm homemade custard.

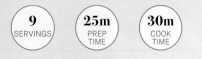

9 SERVINGS | **25m** PREP TIME | **30m** COOK TIME

CALORIES 317 | CARBS 5.4G | FAT 31G | PROTEIN 4.5G

70g (2½oz) unsalted butter, melted

2 large eggs, whisked

1 teaspoon vanilla extract

40g (1½oz) coconut flour (see Tip)

70g (2½oz) powdered erythritol, sifted

1 teaspoon baking powder

For the sauce

90ml (6 tablespoons) double cream

2 tablespoons water

20g (¾oz) powdered erythritol, sifted

2 teaspoons unsalted butter

1 teaspoon vanilla extract

For the custard

250ml (9fl oz) double cream

1 teaspoon vanilla extract

4 large egg yolks

2 tablespoons powdered erythritol, sifted

2 tablespoons ground arrowroot (or use 2 x 8g/¼oz sachets)

Preheat the oven to 200°C/180°C fan/400°F/gas mark 6 and grease and line the base and sides of 15cm (6in) square brownie tin with baking paper.

Let the melted butter cool a little before whisking with the whisked eggs in a bowl. Add the vanilla extract and mix well to combine.

In a separate bowl, combine the coconut flour, erythritol and baking powder. Pour the egg mixture into the dry mixture and stir to combine, working quickly. Pour the mixture into the prepared dish and bake on the lowest rack for 18–20 minutes or until a cake tester inserted into the centre comes out clean (I always rotate the dish halfway through cooking and cover with a sheet of foil for the last 5 minutes).

While the pudding is baking, make the sauce. Simply melt all the elements together in a small saucepan over a low–medium heat and cook for 4–5 minutes.

When the pudding is ready, pierce the surface all over with a fork, then pour the warm sauce over the top to completely soak in. Reduce the oven temperature to 100°C/80°C fan/200°F/gas mark ¼ and return the pudding to the oven to keep warm until you're ready to serve.

To make the custard, combine the double cream and vanilla extract in a non-stick saucepan. Place over a low heat and gently warm through.

In a separate bowl, whisk together the egg yolks, erythritol and arrowroot, ensuring there are no lumps.

Slowly drizzle the warmed cream into the yolk mixture, whisking continuously. This step tempers the eggs. It is important the cream isn't too hot, or it may cook parts of the egg. Once it's all been whisked in, return the whole lot to the saucepan.

Cook over a low–medium heat, whisking continuously with a silicone-tipped whisk for about 7–12 minutes until it has thickened beautifully, being very careful not to let it get too hot (no one wants scrambled-egg custard). Pass the custard through a sieve into a clean bowl or jug.

Slice the warm pudding into 9 equal-sized pieces and serve drizzled with the warm custard. The dessert can be frozen, but should always be eaten warm because the buttery sauce will solidify unpleasantly. After defrosting, gently reheat in a warm oven (120°C/100°C fan/250°F/gas mark ½) for 15–20 minutes. The custard, however, should always be made fresh and served warm for best results.

*

If you prefer to use almond flour, replace the coconut flour with 115g (4oz) almond flour and follow the same method. The almond flour version (pictured) comes in at 5.7g carbs per serving and gives a fluffier texture.

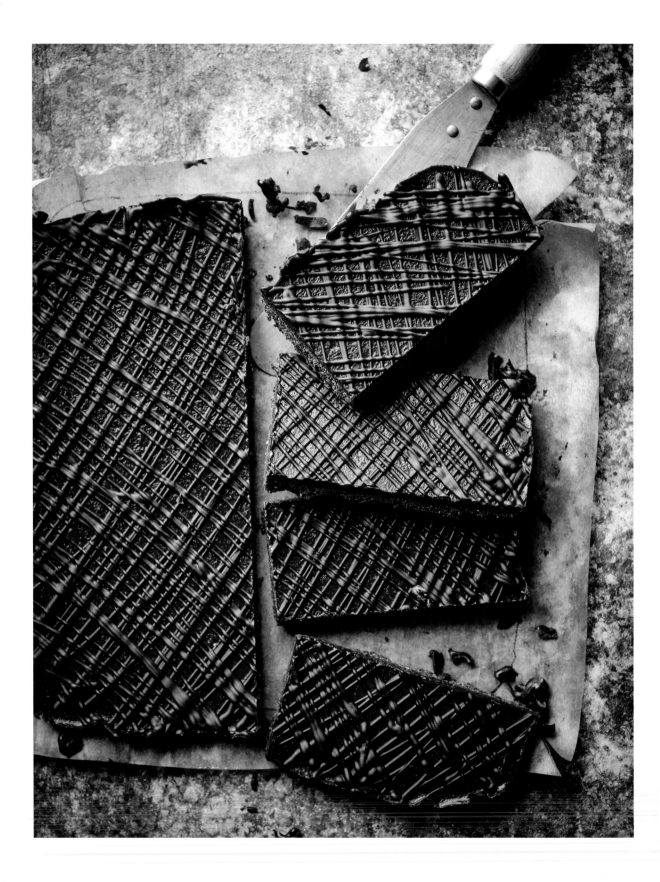

Chocolate Protein Bars

These chocolate bars are a lovely grab-and-go option when you want a sweet treat that boasts a little protein. I use ground chia seeds here, which provide the bulk in these delicious bars, as well as the protein. Chia is also a great source of fibre and omega-3. I decorate them with more melted chocolate, but that is optional (although additional chocolate is never a bad thing!).

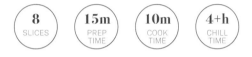

8 SLICES | **15m** PREP TIME | **10m** COOK TIME | **4+h** CHILL TIME

PER SLICE: CALORIES 298 | CARBS 4.5G | FAT 28G | PROTEIN 5.4G

140g (5oz) unflavoured (odourless) coconut oil

100g (3½oz) dark chocolate (85 per cent cocoa), broken into pieces

4–5 drops liquid stevia (optional)

110g (3¾oz) ground (milled) chia seeds

110g (3¾oz) powdered erythritol, sifted

2½ tablespoons unsweetened cocoa powder

For the chocolate drizzle (optional)

50g (1¾oz) dark chocolate (85 per cent cocoa), broken into pieces

2 teaspoons double cream

15g (½oz) unsalted butter

*

I think these are nicest when you remove them from the fridge about 30 minutes before enjoying, but Mark disagrees and loves them straight from the fridge!

Grease and line the base and sides of a 16cm (6¼in) square brownie tin with baking paper.

Very gently melt the coconut oil and chocolate together in a large non-stick saucepan over a low heat, mixing until combined. Add a few drops of liquid stevia (if using).

At the same time, combine the ground chia, erythritol and cocoa powder in a large bowl. Pour the melted coconut chocolate mixture into the bowl and mix everything together to combine. Tip the mixture into the prepared tin and place in the fridge for 3–4 hours until set.

If you choose to make the optional chocolate drizzle topping, place the chocolate, cream and butter in a small non-stick saucepan over a low heat and allow to melt together. It's important to melt them at the same time to avoid a grainy mixture. Leave to cool a little before covering the set bar mixture with the melted chocolate topping. You could also fill a small piping bag (fitted with a small, round-tipped nozzle) and drizzle the chocolate topping over in a decorative pattern, as pictured.

Allow the chocolate drizzle to set completely before slicing the bar mixture into 8 equal-sized mini bars. (If you are skipping the chocolate drizzle, remove the mixture from the fridge 30 minutes before slicing, as this makes it easier to cut.) Wrap each one up individually and keep in the fridge or freezer. To defrost, just leave in the fridge for a few hours.

Cheat's Crème Caramel

For this fantastic crème caramel, I add the 'caramel' element after the dessert sets. I played around with doing it the more conventional way in my trials, but the results were never right. So, I did the obvious thing: I cheated! And the result is well worth my naughty short-cut. Drizzle over whichever sugar-free syrup you have to hand (or leave it out altogether and simply enjoy the decadence of this sweet 'set' custard). *Pictured on page 134.*

4 SERVINGS | **10m** PREP TIME | **50m** COOK TIME | **4+h** SETTING TIME

CALORIES 483 | CARBS 5.3G | FAT 50G | PROTEIN 6.4G

350ml (12fl oz) double cream

150ml (5fl oz) water

1½ teaspoons vanilla extract

100g (3½oz) powdered erythritol, sifted

2–3 drops liquid stevia (optional)

2 large eggs, plus 2 large egg yolks

4 tablespoons sugar-free syrup

salt flakes (optional, see Tip)

Preheat the oven to 180°C/160°C fan/350°F/gas mark 4. Grease 4 ramekins and place inside a deep roasting dish.

Place the cream, water, vanilla, erythritol and liquid stevia (if using) in a non-stick saucepan over a medium heat and bring to a light simmer for 1–2 minutes to warm through.

Meanwhile, in a bowl, whisk together the eggs and egg yolks very well.

Remove the pan of warm cream from the heat and add 7–8 tablespoons of the mixture to the bowl of whisked eggs, adding 1 tablespoon at a time and whisking well between each addition. This tempers the eggs so they don't scramble. Pour the tempered egg mixture into the saucepan with the rest of the cream mixture and return the pan to a low heat. Continue to whisk for 3–4 minutes.

Divide the mixture between the 4 ramekins, then pour boiling water into the roasting dish so that it comes a little more than halfway up the outsides of the ramekins.

Bake on the lowest rack in the oven for 40-45 minutes. I always carefully rotate the dish halfway through.

Very carefully remove the tray from the oven, then remove each ramekin from the hot water and leave to cool on a cooling rack. Once cooled completely, cover each one with clingfilm and keep in the fridge for at least 4 hours (or even overnight, if you decide to make this the day before).

To serve, slide a knife around the edge of each ramekin and gently turn it upside down on to a plate or bowl to release the crème caramel. Drizzle a tablespoon of your favourite sugar-free syrup over each one.

Try adding a tiny pinch of salt flakes on top of the syrup before serving. A little salt actually adds a lovely flavour (and texture) to sweet goods!

Double-layered Jelly

with Simple Cream Finish

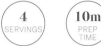

4 SERVINGS   **10m** PREP TIME

285ml (9½fl oz) boiling water

1 single packet sugar-free jelly (11.5g/½oz), flavour of your choice

120ml (4fl oz) double cream

120ml (4fl oz) cold water

For the topping

160ml (5½fl oz) double cream

This cute three-layered dessert is so easy to make: just remember that each layer must set well before the next is added. Gelatine sets when chilled, so keep the second jug of mix at room temperature before pouring. Note: sugar-free jelly powder usually contains aspartame, which is considered 'dirty' keto. *Pictured on pages 134–135.*

CALORIES 327 | CARBS 1.1G | FAT 35G | PROTEIN 1.1G

Pour the boiling water into a jug and whisk in the packet of jelly. Pour exactly half of this mixture into a second jug. Set the second jug aside (at room temperature) for now.

Pour the double cream into the first jug and whisk well to combine. Divide the mixture between 4 serving glasses. Refrigerate for 2–3 hours to completely set.

Once the creamy layer has set, whisk the cold water into the jug set aside earlier, then pour this over the creamy layer. Return to the fridge until the top jelly layer has set.

To serve, simply pour the double cream over the jelly to make the top layer.

Cappuccino Mousse Pots

4 SERVINGS   **10m** PREP TIME   **3+h** SETTING TIME

300ml (10fl oz) double cream

1 teaspoon gelatine powder

3 teaspoons instant coffee granules

1 teaspoon vanilla extract

2 tablespoons powdered erythritol, sifted

ground cinnamon or unsweetened cocoa powder, to dust (optional)

I love the flavour of coffee! These little mouse pots are the one sweet treat I will happily devour. If you have these in the evening, you could use decaf instant coffee. *Pictured on pages 134–135.*

CALORIES 359 | CARBS 2.3G | FAT 38G | PROTEIN 2.6G

Pour 70ml (2¼fl oz) of the cream into a small non-stick saucepan and the remainder into a large mixing bowl. Add the gelatine powder, coffee granules and vanilla to the saucepan and gently warm over a low–medium heat until the coffee and gelatine dissolve. Set aside.

Meanwhile, add the erythritol to the bowl of cream and use a hand mixer to whip to semi-stiff peaks. Pour in the coffee mixture and whip one last time to combine well. Quickly divide the mixture between 4 small pots before leaving to set in the fridge for at least 3 hours. Serve dusted with ground cinnamon or cocoa, if you like.

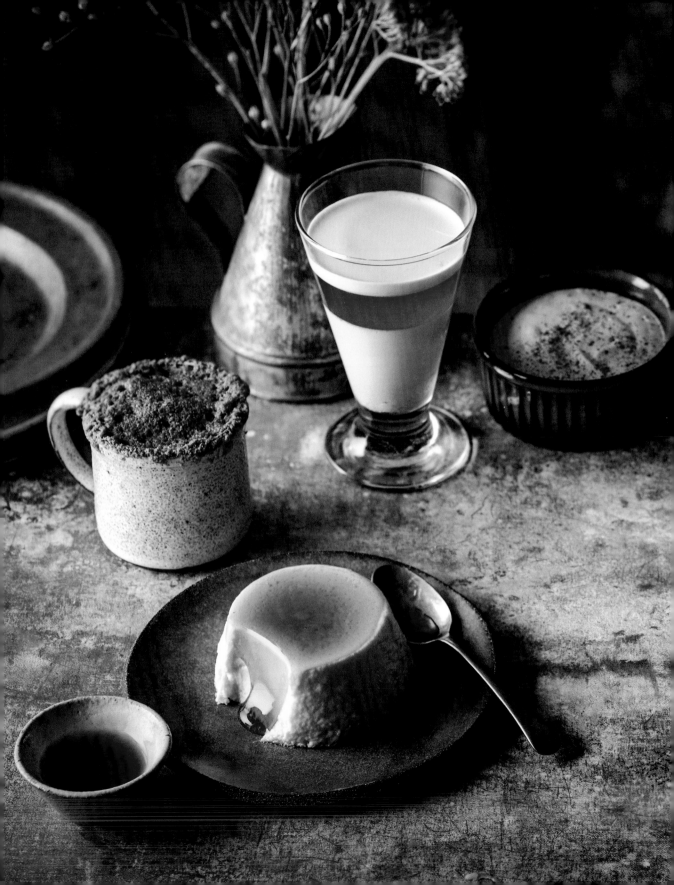

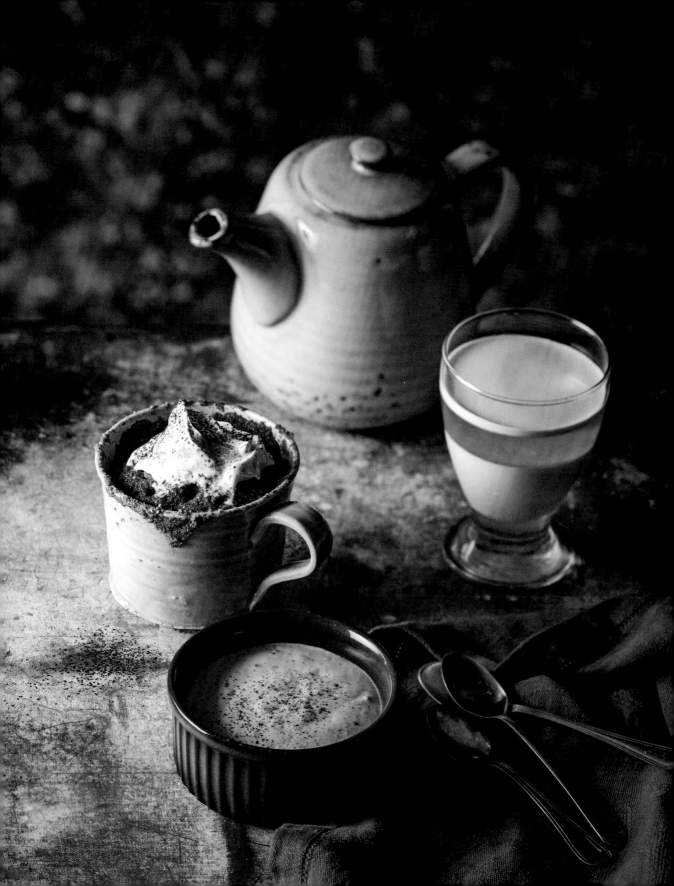

Raspberry Cheesecake Lollies

Creamy and delicious with a sweet, tart element, these raspberry cheesecake lollies are a fabulous way to end your summer lunches when entertaining friends. My husband loves them, so I bet this means the kids will too! Lolly moulds are so easy to find, and they are a great little investment – I use them a lot and have many different and exciting lolly ideas on my blog.

6 LOLLIES   **15m** PREP TIME   **12h** FREEZE TIME

CALORIES 195 | CARBS 3.1G | FAT 18G | PROTEIN 2G

260g (9oz) fresh raspberries

1 teaspoon lemon juice

160ml (5½fl oz) double cream

120g (4¼oz) full-fat cream cheese

2 tablespoons powdered erythritol, sifted

2–3 drops liquid stevia (optional)

Place the raspberries and lemon juice in a mini food processor or food chopper. Blitz to a smooth purée and set aside.

In a large bowl, use a hand mixer to whip the double cream to semi-stiff peaks. Add the cream cheese and erythritol and whip well to evenly combine.

Spoon a little raspberry purée into the bottom of each of the 6 lolly moulds (100ml/3½fl oz) in capacity, then fold the remaining purée through the whipped creamy mixture.

Divide the creamy mixture between the lolly moulds. Since a lot of air has been incorporated into the mixture, you may need to scoop the mixture into each mould slowly, knocking the mould on the kitchen counter to remove air pockets.

Add the lolly sticks, then place in the freezer overnight.

Transfer the lollies to the fridge 30 minutes before eating, or simply run hot water over the outside of the mould to make them easier to slide out.

If you choose not to make lollies, this mixture is equally delicious served in little pots, but leave them in the fridge for at least 2 hours.

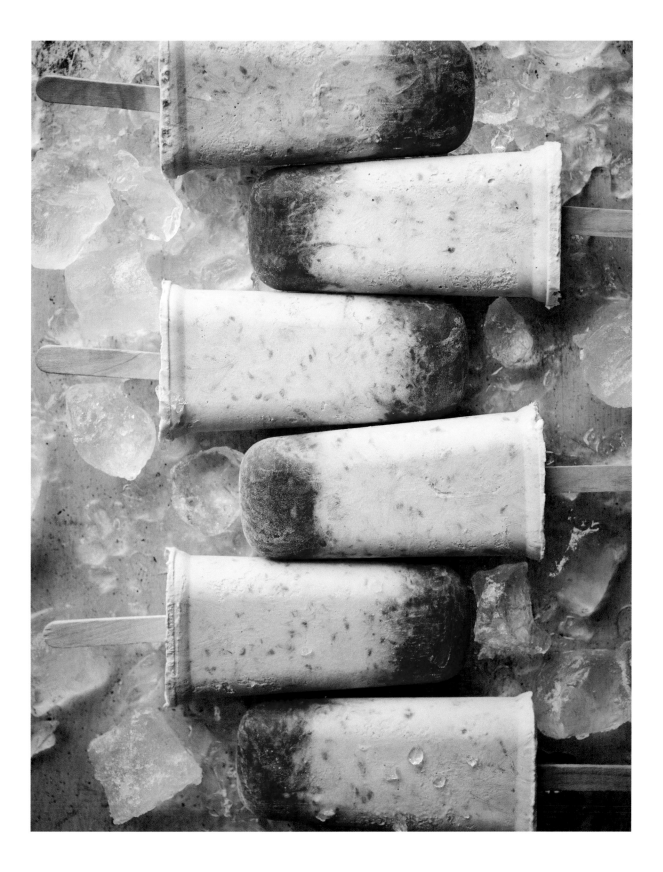

Hot Chocolate

4 SERVINGS   **10m** PREP TIME   **10m** COOK TIME

360ml (12¼fl oz) double cream

360ml (12¼fl oz) tepid water

100g (3½oz) dark chocolate (85 per cent cocoa), broken into pieces

1½ tablespoons unsweetened cocoa powder

1 tablespoon powdered erythritol, sifted

2–3 drops liquid stevia (optional)

unsweetened cocoa powder, to dust (optional)

Who doesn't love a mug of warm hot chocolate? This one is rich and super-chocolatey! Be sure to always melt chocolate over a very low heat to avoid it splitting or going grainy. An indulgent creamy topping is optional, and therefore not included in the macros.

CALORIES 576 | CARBS 8.1G | FAT 58G | PROTEIN 5.3G

Place all the hot chocolate ingredients in a medium-sized saucepan over a very low heat and allow all the elements to melt together and warm through. Once melted, whisk gently to combine. Taste the mixture to check it is suitably hot and sweet.

Divide the hot chocolate between 4 mugs and top with the whipped cream (if using), see Tip. Dust with additional cocoa powder, if you wish.

Strawberry Shakes

4 SERVINGS   **15m** PREP TIME   **5m** COOK TIME   **2+h** CHILL TIME

300g (10½oz) fresh strawberries, roughly chopped

1 teaspoon lemon juice

230ml (8fl oz) unsweetened almond milk

2–3 drops liquid stevia (optional)

300ml (10fl oz) double cream

40g (1½oz) powdered erythritol, sifted

These creamy shakes are the perfect end to a lovely summer meal and the mixture makes enough for 4 small yet decadent shakes. If your macros allow for it, make them even more show-stopping by topping with an optional sweetened whipped cream (see Tip) and more chopped strawberries!

CALORIES 393 | CARBS 6.9G | FAT 39G | PROTEIN 2.1G

Blitz the strawberries and lemon juice in a mini food processor until smooth. Pour half the purée into a small saucepan and cook over a medium heat for 5 minutes. Tip the remaining purée into a bowl and add the almond milk and liquid stevia (if using). Now add the cooked strawberry mixture and use a hand blender to blitz well.

Meanwhile, in a second, larger bowl, use a hand mixer to whip the cream and erythritol to semi-stiff peaks. Pour in the strawberry mixture and whip well to combine. Place in the fridge to chill completely. (If you have an ice-cream maker, you could partially churn the mixture to a thick, milkshake consistency.) Top with sweet whipped cream (if using) and chopped strawberries if you want to.

*

Make a sweet cream
topping by whipping
200ml (7fl oz) double cream
with 2 tablespoons sifted
erythritol until semi-soft
peaks form.

Chocolate Microwave Cakes

These dreamy chocolate mug cakes take just a few minutes to throw together. Here, I used the more inexpensive coconut flour (although I give an option if you have almond flour, see Tip) and the results are perfect. Enjoy them warm with a dollop of extra cream. The texture is fantastic and just like moist cake. Yum! *Pictured on pages 134–135.*

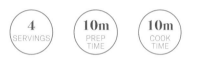

4 SERVINGS | **10m** PREP TIME | **10m** COOK TIME

CALORIES 282 | CARBS 5.9G | FAT 25G | PROTEIN 6.7G

40g (1½oz) unflavoured (odourless) coconut oil, gently melted

2 large eggs

80ml (2¾fl oz) double cream

3 drops liquid stevia (optional)

1 teaspoon vanilla extract

40g (1½oz) coconut flour

1 teaspoon baking powder

70g (2½oz) powdered erythritol, sifted

1 tablespoon unsweetened cocoa powder, plus extra to serve (optional)

whipped cream, to serve (optional)

Grease 4 ramekins or microwave-safe mugs.

Allow the coconut oil to cool slightly before whisking into the eggs in a medium-sized bowl. Add the double cream, vanilla extract and liquid stevia (if using) and whisk well.

In a separate bowl, combine the coconut flour, baking powder, erythritol and cocoa powder. Pour the creamy egg mixture into the dry mixture and mix well to combine. Divide the mixture equally between the 4 ramekins or mugs.

Cooking one at a time, place a ramekin in the centre of the microwave and cook on high for 1 minute 30 seconds. Repeat with the others.

Tip the cakes out of the ramekins (you may need to slide a knife around the edges) and enjoy while they are still warm with some whipped cream and dusted with a little cocoa powder (if desired). Alternatively, just eat them straight from the ramekins (but remember they are hot!).

These cakes are best eaten immediately, but they can be kept in the fridge and reheated in a warm oven (120°C/100°C/250°F/gas mark ½), covered with foil, for 15-20 minutes.

If you prefer to use almond flour, replace the coconut flour with 80g (2¾oz) almond flour and reduce the double cream to only 40ml (1¼fl oz). I have tried and enjoyed both versions. The almond flour version is 5.3g carbs per serving.

Index

Index

UK/US Glossary

Ingredients
celeriac – *celery root*
coriander – *cilantro*
courgette – *zucchini*
dark chocolate – *bittersweet chocolate*
desiccated coconut – *dried shredded coconut*
double cream – *heavy cream*
dried chilli flakes – *dried hot red pepper flakes*
flaked almonds – *slivered almonds*
flat-leaf parsley –*Italian parsley*
minced beef/pork – *ground beef/pork*
pepper (red/yellow) – *bell pepper/capsicum*
prawns – *shrimp*
soured cream – *sour cream*
spring onions – *scallions*
stock – *broth*
tomato purée – *tomato paste*
wild rocket – *wild arugula*

Equipment
baking paper – *parchment paper*
baking tray – *baking sheet*
clingfilm – *plastic wrap*
frying pan – *skillet*
roasting tray – *roasting pan*
sieve – *fine mesh strainer*
tart tin – *tart pan*

Note on eggs
A large egg in the US is slightly different to a large egg in the US. A UK medium egg is closer in size to a US large egg, and a UK large egg is closer in size to a US extra-large egg.

Acknowledgements

To my lovely agent, Clare: thank you from the bottom of my heart for all that you do. You have helped me realise my dreams, and you certainly have not heard the last of my long list of book ideas! (I suspect you will be reading through my next book proposals at the same time as you read this.)

To the dynamic team at Kyle: Judith, Jo, Zakk and Allison, our proofreader Vicky and our designer Nicky – thank you for your hard work and dedication. My fabulous editor, Tara – I am so grateful for your guidance, and I couldn't be more thrilled to have you on my side. I love that we have now smashed out three beautiful books together.

I wouldn't consider any other photographer than the super-talented Maja Smend to bring my food to life. Maja, your patience is endless, and your talented eye is revered. Just like I say to Tara all the time: you are always right, and I trust you implicitly. I only hope you had as much fun as I did on all my books. Thank you also to Morag for selecting the beautiful props – I always love seeing what you have brought to the shoots. To Phoebe, thank you for everything. And to Sam Folan ('Super Sam', as I like to call you!), a huge thanks for everything on our last two shoot days.

To my trusty group of recipe testers, many of whom have been working with me for several years: your role is so crucial to me as a cookbook author: Amanda, Angie, Cindy, Daryl, Ellie, Gabby, Heino, Joanita, Julie, Kim, Olivia, Paul, Pippa, Stella, Sue, and Tanya – thank you all so very much! I am eternally grateful for your time and effort.

Lastly, to my husband, Mark. I must say that I was quite proud of us during the pandemic. Despite how low we felt over that time, we didn't (completely!) lose our minds, and plenty of good things came out of it. I am not referring to this book – I am referring to how much the dogs and I loved having you home, all to ourselves, for more than 18 months. We will miss you terribly as you go back to travelling, but we know that you are doing what you genuinely love, and I understand that more than anyone. This is for you, of course.

– Monya

@mkilianpalmer (Instagram) | www.fatsoflife.co.uk